Dysphagia
Naturally

TIPS, TOOLS &
RESOURCES FOR
PATIENTS WITH
SWALLOWING
DISORDERS

A resource guide for patients and caregivers

JULIA S. TUCHMAN

Dysphagia Naturally: Tips, Tools, and Resources for
Patients with Swallowing Disorders

A Resource Guide for Patients and Caregivers

By Julia S. Tuchman

©2022, Julia S. Tuchman

"In her book, Dysphagia Naturally, Julia delivers a well-curated collection of resources and advice from one dysphagia sufferer to another. Julia's story is not uncommon and it will resonate with many of those who struggle with swallowing disorders or have a loved one who does. From sharing tried and tested recipes and apps, to delivering pragmatic travel recommendations and messages of hope for other patients, Julia leads by example in what building dysphagia advocacy and awareness looks like".

—*Gabi Constantinescu, PhD, Speech-Language Pathologist, Adjunct Assistant Professor, Communication Sciences and Disorders Department, University of Alberta, is a clinician researcher who treats swallowing difficulties*

———————————

"Throughout my many years treating patients rehabilitating from health crises I've become well-acquainted with swallowing disorders (dysphagia) and the feelings of anxiety and helplessness patients experience as to how to proceed. Julia Tuchman's Dysphagia Naturally is a wellspring of information and resources that will engender hope and a renewed sense of control in dealing with the challenges dysphagia presents."

–*Margaret M. Eaton, Psy.D. Psychologist*

———————————

"Julia's comprehensive and easy-to-read book is a gem! It is a true guide full of resources and hope for anyone looking to move forward in the healthiest way possible."

–*Amy B. Scher, author of* This Is How I Save My Life *and* How To Heal Yourself When No One Else Can

"Julia Tuchman's Dysphagia Naturally is the long-awaited book that has been missing from the field of dysphagia. Not only has Ms. Tuchman compiled and systematically organized an extensive list of valuable resources, but her story will be familiar and ring true to sufferers of dysphagia and their caregivers. After living with dysphagia for over 25 years, Julia has keen insight into the day-to-day struggle of living with swallowing difficulties, and she openly shares what she has learned. She outlines various recipes, food sources, equipment, and practical recommendations with a wonderful sense of humor that is sure to provide much needed compassion and assistance for others with dysphagic disorders."

—Teresa Ashman, PhD, ABPP, Associate Professor, NYU Langone Medical Center, Rusk Rehabilitation and Hackensack Meridian, JFK Johnson Rehabilitation. Dr. Ashman is a clinical rehabilitation neuropsychologist with over 20 years of research and clinical experience treating people with chronic health conditions.

"I just finished reading Dysphagia Naturally. I am in awe of you Julia, and all the contributors in this book. It is going to be a life-changer for not only dysphagia sufferers, but medical professionals, caregivers and family and friends. It's been written as a guide for dysphagia but I also feel it will be a must-have in everybody's toolbox for survival. This resource book will be so helpful for so many out there."

—Sally Gillipse , dysphagia patient, New Zealand.

Contents

Why I wrote this resource book

In all my years of living with dysphagia, I have never seen any book or resource guide created by a patient for other patients with this condition. I've seen recipe books for patients and medical books created for swallowing therapists, but no resource self-help guide for patients.

Over the last year, I have noticed how many new people were joining dysphagia support groups on Facebook seeking help on how to adjust and live with this debilitating disorder. These groups consisted of patients who gave support and tips to other patients. Many complained how they were given no instructions by their doctor, and were looking for support and tips. Because I have lived with a swallowing disorder since 1995, I just assumed most of my knowledge of how to survive with this was common sense or common knowledge. However, I have learned that this is not true.

This summer, my mother had a choking episode after a long illness. For a few months, she had to eat soft and dysphagia-safe foods. I thought her medical aides would know what to do. I was shocked when I saw that one of them had given her a bowl that contained very thick oatmeal—so thick it was like glue. Even someone without a swallowing issue would have had trouble getting the cement-like mixture down. Because she said she could not swallow it, my mother just left it uneaten. When I tried to explain to the aide that this was not safe, she had a very confused look on her face. I even put it back in the blender to show her she would have to add much more water to make it thinner in order for my mom to safely eat it.

Another aide left whole fruit by her bed, which was a choking hazard. When I tried to explain the same to her how this was dangerous, she too had the same perplexed look. A light bulb went off in my head: This is not common knowledge. People do not know how to make foods for people with swallowing disorders—not even medical aides, who are supposedly trained. The reason I had just thought it was common knowledge is because it was just natural to me or came "naturally" to me. I had had to eat like this for so many years it was just part of my life—as common as knowing how to brush my teeth or wash my face.

There are a few companies I have listed in this book that were created because the founders saw that a product such as theirs did not exist for people with dysphagia. One was a doctor who, when ill with cancer, realized there were no healthy nutritional shake alternatives with no chemicals or other unhealthy ingredients. A woman whose father suffered from an illness, and had to be tube fed created another company. She was horrified to see how unhealthy the feeding tube concoctions were, and that no other healthy options were available. She created an entire company supplying organic functional formulas that are pure whole nutrition without chemicals because she wanted a healthy option for her dad that would also aid in his healing. Necessity truly is the mother of invention. Because there are no resource guides for this disorder, I decided to create one myself. This is the guide I wish someone had given me when I was first diagnosed with dysphagia.

My Story

In 1988, during my college years, I contracted mononucleosis. I expected to be well enough in a few months to return to school and "normal" life, but that never happened. Many months later, I was still ill and was later diagnosed as having post-viral Myalgic Encephalomyelitis/chronic fatigue syndrome (ME/CFS). It remains a misunderstood illness, but in those days, even less was known about it. It felt as if I had the flu every day. With brain fog and extreme exhaustion, there was very little I could do. I was now disabled and often bedridden. A five-year relationship with my first love ended, as did many friendships. It was devastating and confusing. It felt like I had fallen down a rabbit hole, and I had to figure out how to find my way out. I did the best I could, and along the way found a number of holistically trained doctors to help me.

A few years later, I woke up one morning unable to swallow solid food. Because I had such severe environmental and food allergies at the time due to this illness, I just assumed it was an allergic reaction and would improve. It did not. I was now barely getting down liquids, and was becoming malnourished. When I went to the local hospital, they did a modified barium swallow study (MBSS) and other swallow tests. The tests showed I had a severe swallow dysfunction. I had no initiation of a swallow, and food would get stuck in the esophagus. Peristalsis was almost non-existent. The doctor was alarmed and sent me for testing with a neurologist. He thought I might have ALS (Lou Gehrig's disease) or another neurological illness and wanted to rule those out, as it was rare to have this at such a young age. The neurologist could not make a definitive diagnosis and had no answers as to why my swallow was so impaired. They knew I had neurological damage, but with no diagnoses or cure, I was sent home and had

9

to figure it out all by myself. The doctor did not even send me to a swallow therapist, and I had no idea they even existed. If I had, I would have demanded that help. My mother was making me chicken broth, but I was losing weight fast and felt weak from lack of food. There was no Internet then and there were no support groups to guide me.

Years later, doctors told me it was likely that I had brain and nerve damage due to a virus or mold injury. They also found many autoimmune issues. Nobody really had a definitive answer. I also had severe food sensitivities, so I could not rely on the solutions that other dysphagia patients had discovered. The nutritional drinks Ensure and Boost contained ingredients I could not tolerate due to allergies and sensitivity to food additives and corn syrup. A few years earlier, I met with Dr. Nicholas Gonzales, a specialist who used Dr. William Kelly's protocol for curing cancer and other degenerative diseases. From him, I learned the importance of eating organically, juicing, and other nutritional support. I had always had an interest in holistic medicine and natural healing, and I used that knowledge to begin to figure out how to get adequate healthy organic nutrition. I knew I could not rely on the drinks the hospital supplied to dysphagia patients, and so I had to figure it out for myself. I had no choice. It was not easy, and it was a long learning process.

My hope is that this resource book can help you or your loved one during this difficult journey of living with a swallowing disorder. You do not have to figure it out alone, as I did. There is much more support available now than there was years ago.

> "The first step to healing is to take responsibility for your life. We do not get to choose what happens to us; however, we do have the ability to choose how we respond."
>
> —Dr. Darren Weissman

Swallowing therapists are also referred to as a Speech and Language Pathologist or SLP. They are all one and the same. Not all Speech Language Pathologists are trained to treat swallowing disorders. There are SLPs who do specialize in swallowing and have been trained to assess, diagnose and treat patients with speech and or swallowing disorders. I will use the term swallowing therapist in this book as that is what my own doctor referred to them as and what I have always called these professionals. When you are diagnosed with dysphagia, you will be sent to a SLP who specializes in swallowing. If you are not, then ask to be referred to one.

The Dysphagia Basics

The prevalence of dysphagia is unknown, but epidemiologic studies indicate that the numbers may be as high as 22% of the population over 50 years of age. Several studies conclude that between 300,000 and 600,000 individuals in the United States are affected by neurogenic dysphagia each year. Plus, 10 million Americans are evaluated each year for swallowing difficulties. Because this disorder cuts across so many diseases, dysphagia is poorly understood and often under diagnosed.

Dysphagia symptoms

Each person is different, but some of the common symptoms of this disorder are as follows:

- Coughing during or right after eating or drinking.

- Wet or gurgly sounding voice during or after eating or drinking; extra effort or time needed to chew or swallow.

- Food or liquid leaking from the mouth or getting stuck in the mouth.

- Recurring pneumonia or chest congestion after eating.

- Weight loss or dehydration from not being able to eat enough.

Diagnostic tests for dysphagia

These tests are generally performed by a speech-language pathologist. The most commonly used tests are:

- Modified barium swallow study: the patient eats or drinks food or liquid with barium in it and the swallowing process is viewed on an x-ray.

- Endoscope assessment: using a lighted scope inserted through the nose, allowing the swallow to be viewed on a screen.

- Dysphagia treatment: Treatment depends on the cause, symptoms, and type of swallowing problem. A speech-language pathologist may recommend a specific swallowing treatment (e.g., exercises to improve muscle movement). Positions or strategies to help the individual swallow more effectively specific food and liquid textures that are easier and safer to swallow.

(Dysphagia basics courtesy of the National Foundation of Swallow Disorders. Used with their permission.)

If you have not been seen by a doctor or had a swallow study, I suggest that you do so you know what foods are safe for you, and they can send you to a swallowing therapist who will be able to help you further. This book is to be used as a resource for information and links related to dysphagia. The Swallowing Foundation website offers support and doctor referrals.

swallowingdisorderfoundation.com

The Number One Tip and Tool

The number one piece of advice I have given to people that has helped the most is get a Vitamix blender. Really? you ask. I bought this book to be told to buy a blender? "Aha," as they say on the old commercials from my youth, "not just any blender!" This was the blender that saved my life.

First, I must say, I do not work for Vitamix. I wish I did, as I have told so many dysphagia sufferers to get it that I should work for them. Since the mid-'90s, when I got this blender, it is the number one tool that helped save my life. Yes, it saved my life. This high-speed blender was able to liquefy any food, including all my vitamins and tablets. My swallow was so bad then that I could only get down very thin liquids with no lumps. The Vitamix was powerful enough to make that a possibility. The Vitamix will also make whole juices and soups. Whole juice is different from juice in a juicer as it contains all the fiber too. Nothing is wasted.

A year ago, a woman named Ilanit from Israel, wrote a post on a dysphagia support Facebook page that caught my eye. She was asking for help as she had to strain all her food through a cheesecloth and strainer and the consistency was not correct or safe to swallow. She was hungry and desperate for some support and advice. I advised her to get a Vitamix, but she was hesitant and understandably so. The Vitamix is expensive but even more so in Israel. I told her that for her to get proper nutrition, it would be worth it. She finally did buy it. I smiled reading her thank you note to me. She wrote telling me it saved her life, and she no longer felt hungry. In the ensuing months, I would often see her writing in response to a new member asking for help. She would tell them to get a Vitamix and that it saved her life. Again, it also showed me that what I have learned these many years was not just "known" or common knowledge. I realized I had information that could be helpful to others just diagnosed with this disorder. I am grateful that Ilanit was helped by this information. When I asked her how she felt the Vitamix helped her, she wrote back, saying, "it has really changed my life, and probably saved my life. It did save my life." I understood what she meant. This important tool had saved my life too.

There are other high-power blenders that are less expensive. If you are unable to get a Vitamix, then get the one you can get. I have heard others talk about the Ninja or the new heater blenders that cook as well as blend. I can only vouch for the Vitamix, as I have used this brand for more than 20 years. They have never broken and the only time it did break was when I left a metal spoon in it by mistake and turned the power on. I do not suggest you do that. They do sell refurbished Vitamix blenders on their site that are less expensive.

The Vitamix comes with a recipe and instruction book. With dysphagia, everyone is unique. Like me, the woman from Israel needed liquified foods. Some people need thickeners put in liquids in order to swallow it. Liquids are unsafe for them. There are many levels of dysphagia, so when you do get your Vitamix or other high-powered blender, make sure you know from your doctor what consistency is safe for you or your loved one. Only the swallowing therapist and doctor can tell you what level of dysphagia you are at and what is safe for you. Vitamix can create foods for all levels of dysphagia. Also, it is available from dealers in most countries. Get in contact with Vitamix for more information on dealers in other countries if you are outside of the United States. There are also some countries like India where Vitamix is not available. Look for other high-speed blenders in cases where Vitamix is unavailable or not in your budget.

You will occasionally find sales on the Vitamix web site. If you are looking to take advantage of a payment plan, try QVC. For greater cost savings, check out refurbished mixers offered on the Vitamix web site. One dysphagia patient said she had gotten a reconditioned model ten years ago and it still works great. They also sell an immersion blender that is a hand-held blender for a very reasonable price. Other companies also have hand-held blenders and I have talked to other dysphagia patients or caregivers who use this option.

One dysphagia patient, Sally, wrote me after buying a Vitamix at my recommendation: "Got a Vitamix this weekend. Wow. It is a Rolls Royce of blenders! Can't imagine how I did it before. Thank you for the advice!"

"I can't speak of other high-quality blenders, but my Vitamix has been a life saver! I need completely smooth purees, and I haven't found a food yet that it hasn't been able to handle. Plus, it has a long warranty that the company actually honors!"

—Christina, dysphagia patient

Another blender recommended by some other patients is the Ninja Professional Plus Blender with Auto-IQ. If the Vitamix is too expensive, this one is much cheaper and is another option. One dysphagia patient told me she loves the Pampered Chef cooking blender. There are other high-speed blenders available too, and a simple search on the Internet will give you more options. Vitamix is not the only choice. When I got ill, the Vitamix really was the only high-speed blender available.

"If you can't afford a Vitamix, the Ninja Professional blender is fantastic. I have both and use this one a lot. I haven't been able to tell the difference yet."

—Julie M., dysphagia patient

*Julia's Vitamix cleaning tips: Clean the Vitamix out right away, as it is very easy to do. If you let it sit with some foodstuffs left over, it takes more energy and effort to clean. Because energy is an issue with me, I found this helpful. Also, if the container starts to get discolored, put in half white vinegar, half hot water, and run the blender at high speed for a few minutes. You will find this helps. Be careful when you use hot liquids. Make sure the lid is always tightly secured.

The Vitamix website:

www.vitamix.com

Protein Powders – For Use in Healthy Shakes

Protein powders are an easy and healthy way to add protein and calories to any shake or puree. Protein is essential for good health. Below is a list of protein powders and supplements to add to shakes.

Brands I use

Jay Robb protein powder
Egg and whey flavors

SP Complete by Standard Process
Dairy and non-dairy (I use the rice-based ones but the whey version is just as good.)

Orgain Powder
This brand was created by a doctor, and it carries protein powder that can be used in shakes. I have only used their pre-made shakes, but I have been told that the powders are delicious and their site offers many varieties to choose from. The above powders are the ones I use. I have added an extensive list of others used by dysphagia patients.
orgain.com

Recommendations By other dysphagia patients:

Metagenics Ultrameal Advanced Protein
Metagenics has a wide variety of medical food powders and supplements.
metagenics.com

DysphagiaAide Vanilla Nutrition Shake
290-calorie powder. (Available on Amazon.)

Vital Proteins collagen peptides
Two scoops = 18 grams of protein.

American Natural Superfood All-in-One Protein 'N' Greens

Sevenhills Organic Hemp Powder

Nature's Bounty Optimal Solutions® Complete Protein & Vitamin Shake

Almond Pro
Very high in protein.
facebook.com/almondpro

Grass Fed Pasture Raised Collagen Peptides

Naked Nutrition-Naked Vegan Mass – Natural Vegan Weight Gainer Protein Powder
Good for weight gain. 1,230 calories; 51 grams of protein
nakednutrition.net/products/vegan-weight-gainer

Sunwarrior – Warrior Blend Organic protein powder
sunwarrior.com/products/organic-warrior-blend-vegan-protein-powder

Naked Nutrition protein powders
(Lower caloric options available)
https://nakednutrition.com/collections/protein-powder

Nature's Way (Enzymatic Therapy) Fatigued to Fantastic!™ Energy Revitalization System™
naturesway.com/products/fatigued-to-fantastic-energy-revitalization-system

LiquaCel Liquid Protein
16 Grams of protein and 2.5 grams of arginine. This is a protein supplement that is often recommended by doctors for nutritional help

for patients with medical issues. Consume alone or mix into foods.

* Allergy Research Group Free Aminos
I have included this supplement as it is one that I noticed immediate results with. My chiropractor, who is also a nutritionist, told me I was not getting enough protein and he suggested I buy these. This provides 17 freeform amino acids, including nine essential amino acids. I open the capsule and empty the powder into my almond milk or shake. I did feel more energy and a feeling of well-being. When we eat protein the body has to go through a lot of work to break down the protein to reach the amino acids. Free Aminos are an immediate source of these important aminos. It was true that I had not been taking enough protein when he suggested this. Also, if one has digestive issues, this may be the perfect way to get aminos. Allergy Research Group make doctor formulated formulas. There are other companies that make free form amino supplements. Please check with your own doctor, SLP or nutritionist to ask if these amino acids would be helpful for you or your loved one. They can be added to your shake or puree if needed.

There are so many protein powders and supplement powders on the market, including high calorie ones, if you need to gain weight. Health food stores usually have a wide variety of protein powders for sale in their vitamin sections. There has been a major increase in variety since I was first diagnosed. On a recent trip to my local health food store, I overheard a woman asking the salesperson what protein powder would be best for her husband, who was now on a liquified diet. He brought her the Metagenics Ultrameal powder, saying it was what he recommends. I have used their products in the past, and it is a well-known company.

It is possible to have too much protein, so I do suggest you talk to a health professional to make sure you are not having too little protein, but also that you are not taking too much. It may seem odd to even have to write this as with dysphagia the common issue is trying to get enough nutrition. The truth is anything can be too much. At one time my vitamin D levels were low and I was taking 5,000 IU. My doctor told me that I should not take more than that, so he could not raise my dose. Then when my blood tests showed my D was a bit high for the first time, he lowered the D to 1000. Too much D can be dangerous. It would be very rare to get too much protein, but I feel it is necessary to mention this in the chapter about protein powders because someone with dysphagia might be relying fully on protein powder for their protein source. Check with your doctor or nutritionist to make sure your vitamin and protein levels are safe and beneficial. If the powder has added nutrients, also make sure there is not excess Vitamin D for the day or other nutrients that can be problematic when taken in large doses.

Extra tips

Protein powders can also be added to puree, baby foods or any other food to add more protein. Many caregivers have reported doing this.

The Provale cup
A cup designed by speech-language pathologists (SLPs) for people with dysphagia. The Provale Cup allows for only small swallows at a time.

Thanks goes to hundreds of speech language pathologists and occupational therapists for their help in the design of the Provale® Cup. It allows the patient to have small sips of thin liquid when there are issues with aspirating. You can find this cup on many sites, including Amazon. This is very useful for patients with dementia and dysphagia. A swallow therapist will tell patients who need smaller sips to get this. If you feel this would help you or your loved one, you can ask your doctor or swallow therapist if they feel the Provale cup would be beneficial.

My Vitamix Concoctions
I am sharing my own quick, go-to favorites that I have used during

these many years with dysphagia. I am not a cook, so my simple recipes are just that—simple. I have been amazed at the creativity of the food creations made by other dysphagia patients and caregivers. In this resource book, I have included a list of many support groups. You will find that others share their recipes there as well.

Julia's simple go-to shake full of dense nutrition:

- SP Complete Protein Powder, two scoops (or one scoop of Jay Robb Egg powder)

- One frozen banana

- Frozen blueberries (Cascadian Farms)

- One tablespoon of almond butter (any nut butter will work). If you need more calories add two to three tablespoons.

- One teaspoon of flax seeds, finely ground, or flax oil

- Pinch of stevia sweetener powder (not needed if using Jay Robb Powder as sweetener is already added to that). Add water or almond milk and run on high until it is liquified. It is best to add less rather then more liquid to begin with. You can always add more if it is too thick. It is a learning process for everyone.

I open up all my vitamin capsules and put in the powder. The vitamin tablets I put in whole and they liquify when blended. People have often asked how to take their vitamins when they have swallowing issues. I also add powdered probiotic to my shakes. There are a few vitamin capsules that should not be opened, but most can be. Call the company or ask your doctor. I do know Thorne Research advises against opening their digestive enzymes since they can burn the throat. All of their other vitamins can be dissolved in liquid. The vitamin tablets I have I put in whole and the Vitamix liquifies them with the shake. Make sure to run the blender long enough to do this.

Whole juice in the Vitamix

Peel a cucumber and an apple (remove the core). Put cucumber and apple pieces in the blender. Add water and mix for a few minutes at high level until it is liquified. In one drink, I have the whole nutrition of these two healthy foods. I also use celery for a refreshing and healthy celery juice. You can use any vegetable or fruit as long as you remove the pit, seeds, or stems.

With the whole juice made in the Vitamix, you may need to strain it, based on your level of dysphagia. A chinois, a very fine strainer, is perfect for use with dysphagia if this is a concern. If you are able to get a juicer and are okay with liquids, then a juicer would be a helpful addition. It produces concentrated nutrition that is very thin. The fiber is left behind, so there is no need to use a strainer.

Soups – my go-to for nutritional meals

As long as the soup ingredients do not have any bones, you can make it into a smooth puree at any level of dysphagia in the Vitamix. Add more water for a thinner soup and less water for a thicker soup.

This week, I made an asparagus, potato, onion, and garlic soup and then blended it in the blender. I put the leftover soup in a Mason jar in the fridge, and it lasts me a couple of days. I find if I add chicken to soups, it does come out very smooth and edible. I have heard others say it is more difficult with red meat and more gritty meats, but can be done. You will experiment in the process of creating your own healthy foods and will find out what works for you.

Oatmeal

I put oatmeal through the Vitamix, with added water. This is what I had to teach my mom's health-care aide in order to make the oatmeal safe for my mom to eat. I like to add frozen blueberries or apple slices when preparing it. This adds taste and much needed nutritional value. Cinnamon may be added for taste and has the additional benefit of balancing blood sugar. When putting it through the Vitamix, be mindful of using the right amount of water for safe consumption. But, do not add too much at first or it may become too runny! You can water it down more if you find it is too thick.

Avocado

Put the fruit of the avocado into the blender and add a little water. It becomes a simple avocado pudding that is very healthy. It is a quick two- ingredient recipe that I have used through the years. Many dysphagia patients also add avocado to their shakes for supplemental nutrition and more calorie intake needs. Others add sweetener and chocolate powder to make it into a chocolate pudding.

Freezer pop molds

I make my own freezer pops. You, too, can create very nutritious pops, unlike those that are sold in the store. I have made them out of the protein shake and also from fruit juice. I have heard from other dysphagia patients that creating their own popsicles when their swallow issues were at their worst helped them immensely. One woman said she poured Ensure into molds, and it was the only way to get nutrition after her surgery. Other people created their own healthy shake, then made it into pops. You can even make healthy veggie or fruit pops by making whole juice in the Vitamix and pouring it into the ice mold. I buy concentrated blueberry juice from the health food store and make popsicles out of it by adding water and freezing. I do the same with concentrated lemon juice. With the lemon juice, I do add a pinch of stevia to sweeten it a bit.

There are molds available for pureed foods on Amazon and other websites. I have been amazed at the creations people make for people with dysphagia using these molds. They put the pureed food into the shape of the molds and make the eating experience much more enjoyable. There are also baby food freezer trays that would be helpful when freezing purees. Again, I am amazed at how many more resources and products there are now as compared to years ago.

When I told a friend about some of the foods I make in the Vitamix, she told me it seemed I got more nutrition than she did, and she ate solid foods. She may have been right. Even with dysphagia, we can actually create a very healthy and healing diet. Again, because everyone has a different form of dysphagia and can only deal with different consistencies, talk to your doctor and swallowing therapist. Some people need thickeners that will be given to you so you can drink liquids. I was always okay with liquids. If you do need thickeners, your swallowing therapist or doctor can help you to figure out how to incorporate this into your own Vitamix creations. What is most important is that it is safe for you to swallow. The one thing I hear from so many dysphagia patients I talk to is that you learn what works for you in this process. I agree.

Dysphagia Food Resources

Packaged foods for home or on the go.

Orgain
This company makes delicious premade protein shakes in single-serving carton containers. They offer both milk-based and plant-based options. Orgain was developed by Dr. Andrew Abraham, an integrative medicine specialist, cancer survivor, and self-proclaimed kitchen chemist. Throughout treatment for cancer, Andrew saw a need for a nutritional shake made from all-natural, food-based ingredients and took it upon himself to be the first to make it. Orgain products are a staple for me, and I am very grateful for them as I tolerate them well. I wish Orgain had been in existence when I first got this disorder. It has made my life much easier. I am able to take the company's products with me if I am away for the day and now I do not have to worry about being hungry or left without nutrition.

orgain.com

Kate Farms
A calorically dense, peptide-based nutritional formula made for sole-source or supplemental nutrition for drinking or tube feeding.

katefarms.com

Owyn Complete Meal Protein shakes
They are a vegan alternative that a few patients have told me they use. They come in many flavors, including chocolate, vanilla and strawberry banana. 20 grams of protein. Contains Omega 3 and green superfoods. True health on the go.

Baby foods

I have used organic baby foods in glass containers and in the pouch, in the house and on the go. I enjoy the winter squash by Earth's Best, but there are so many brands and varieties available now. If you need to add liquid to make it okay for you, then empty the food into a cup and add water. Again, ask your doctor first what is safe. Some of the various brands available are Plum Organic Baby Foods, Serenity Kids, Toddler Purees with Bone Broth, and Earth's Best. These have been helpful when traveling or even just out for a few hours. I have brought them to restaurants too. I do know other dysphagia patients and caregivers who make their own fresh baby foods in a Vitamix or other high-speed blenders. They then often freeze the results for later use. There are many baby food makers available online. They both steam the veggies then puree it. This is helpful to make a quick puree and you can then add more water if needed. Many different, favorably reviewed brands are easily discoverable on Amazon.

Noka

Super food smoothies. They have various flavors. I have used the cherry Acai version, and it is very good. Do a Google search, and you will find many brands of smoothies like this that are in a pouch so you can travel with it.

nokaorganics.com

EATBar

A delicious, gluten-free bar that melts in your mouth for people who need food that is easier to swallow. Created by a speech pathologist, it does have a high level of sugar, so if you are diabetic, this will not be for you. I did write to the company, and they told me they are working on a low-sugar alternative. I look forward to that.

theeatbar.com

Trace Minerals Research Electrolyte Stamina Power Pak

This product includes the Electrolyte Replacement & Immune Support

Drink, with the following:

1,200 mg Vitamin C-B Vitamins
Electrolytes
Antioxidants
Ionic Trace Minerals
Low Sugar Non-GMO
Certified Vegan

This drink has helped me greatly and is very easy to travel with. I add it to water. You can add it to shakes or add thickener if liquids are an issue.

USDA Organic Purathick

A tasteless organic thickener, this thickens hot and cold liquids for people with dysphagia. Rave reviews because it does not change the taste of foods as so many other products do.

Canned soups

Canned soups were what I traveled with and have always been helpful as a quick meal. I have used Amy's Kitchen Soups because they are healthy and natural. Amy's Lentil Soup was and has been my go-to as I have always been able to tolerate it allergy-wise, but there are so many other choices to suit one's taste. Any canned soup or canned foods like ravioli can be made into a puree or even thinner using a high-speed blender.

Applesauce

Vermont Village makes an unsweetened organic applesauce in sealed single-size containers that are easy to take with you. They come in different flavors. My favorite is the apple and cinnamon. Other companies also make applesauce, so pick your favorite and check the ingredients for healthy options.

GOGO squeeZ foods

I found these in the regular grocery store. They have yogurt smoothies with fruit in pouches for on the go. There are also fruit and veggie mixes in pouches. Many are organic and all natural. They need to be in the fridge after you open the individual pouches, so they are perfect for travel or out for the day.

www.gogosqueez.com

Powdered peanut butter

This is an alternative way to add peanut flavor to foods without increasing the risk of choking. It adds protein and fiber and can be mixed with other foods or added to smoothies or drinks. For those allergic to peanuts, there are companies that have powdered almond butter (e.g., Barney Butter Powdered Almond Butter). I add fine flax powder as well as flax oil to my shakes for extra fiber. Remember, oils are a good way to get needed nutrition in your purees and smoothies. They also sell individual packets of nut butters, which are great for on-the-go or travel.

Pacific Foods (broth and stocks)

Pacific Foods makes organic chicken broth, vegetable broth, and bone broths that they sell as personal-size portions that can be taken with you. They can also be added to soups or purees you make to provide flavor and nutrition.

pacificfoods.com/our-products/broths-and-stocks

Protein nutrition shakes

Popular brands include Ensure and Boost, but more are available. If you do well with them, and they are helpful, then use them. In researching this book, I found that Boost has a very high calorie version to help with weight gain (over 500 calories). Another patient who needed to gain weight uses Scandishake which has 580 calories per serving. In this book, I have tried to provide more natural alternatives, but I am also of the mind to use whatever works for you. My mother loved Ensure, and it helped her greatly. Ensure and Boost also offer puddings that are high in nutrition and calories. A parent of a child with dysphagia recommended PediaSure Peptide Shakes for kids and told me these have been a lifesaver for her child. Ensure Glucerna is used by a caregiver for her father who has both dysphagia and diabetes. It is good to know that there is an alternative available for patients who have both diabetes and dysphagia.

Again, a simple online search will lead you to sites that sell these. So remember, use what works for you and what your doctor agrees is safe for you. You are the best judge of what you like taste-wise as well as nutritionally. It is important to get enough nutrition and calories while living with dysphagia.

Some people put a protein bar they enjoy in the shake through the Vitamix to add even more calories and nutrition when needed. I recently discovered a high protein (8 grams) cottage cheese bar by Spēka that I recommend. Children's hospitals have been interested in it as it is good-tasting and softer with a lot of protein. They can be kept frozen for 18 months and it is a pure product with no preservatives. Make sure to thaw it before you add to the shake or eat.
spekabar.com

Most any protein bar can be fed through a high-speed blender, adding flavor, protein, and calories to any shake. If you are a caretaker, make sure it is smooth when done with no bits or pieces and safe to consume for the level of dysphagia. To be extra safe, consider also using a strainer.

I eat dark chocolate and let it melt in my mouth. Confession: I may very well eat too much dark chocolate! You will find what works for you and what you can safely swallow as you go along. Many people with dysphagia tell me that finding what works for them is a learning process. They work with their swallowing therapist and doctors, but it is the patient who ultimately has to decide what works best for them. I found I was able to eat toast with butter if I took a bite of the toast and got it down with the soup. Others in the dysphagia support groups will share their own tricks and options that they are able to use. One woman uses a vegan cheese sauce on her soups. I am thinking of trying to melt Go Veggie brand cheese on my soup now because of her suggestion. I made some very well-cooked pureed consistency Lundeberg rice pasta and added a few slices of the Go Veggie's cheese on it. The result was a dysphagia version of mac and cheese that worked for me. The help of others in these support groups is invaluable as everyone shares their creations and recipes.

*Dysphagia airplane travel tip
If you have been diagnosed with dysphagia and are traveling by plane, contact the airline about their rules for taking food and drink onto the plane with you. In the past, with a note from my doctor, I was able to board with my special foods.

Also, portable blenders are now available. These can make a day out easier, as well as enable you to spend longer periods of time away from home. Portable blenders are inexpensive and like everything else, can be found online. I have heard from patients who bring the portable blenders to restaurants so they can blend their food there.

For more detailed instructions for travel with dysphagia, please visit the following link on the essential puree page listed below:
essentialpuree.com/travel-tips-dysphagia-patient

Pre-made dysphagia meals (delivery)

Savor ease
"The mission behind Savorease is to improve the dining health for those on a restricted diet. Whether you are 1 or 99 years old, it is a shareable, nutritious small meal. We are proud of the unique crunch of our crackers before they melt in the mouth, and the delicious flavors of all of the products that bring back positive eating memories for you to enjoy."
savorease.com

Blossom Foods
blossomfoods.com

Gourmet Pureed
gourmetpureed.com

Once Upon a Farm
onceuponafarmorganics.com

Mom's Meals
www.momsmeals.com

Hormel Health Labs
Hormel has many foods for people with dysphagia. They also have pureed meal kits with pre-made pureed meals. Ingredients are listed on the site. Many different options and meals are offered.
hormelhealthlabs.com

Home Health Nutrition
When you get to the site, click on Conditions, then Dysphagia. They list many dysphagia food offerings. Look up the Café Puree section of their site. You will find many purees in the shape of the original foods
hhnutrition.com

Thick-It Purees
Canned puree meals for dysphagia patients.
thickit.com

*If you are in a country other than the US, search online for resources in your area. Here are a couple of stand-out international dysphagia food delivery services to whet your appetite:

Australia
Care Food Company
carefoodco.com.au

United Kingdom
It's Made for You Softer Foods from Oakhouse Foods
itsmadeforyou.co.uk

Feeding Tube Resources

Natural feeding tube formulas

Functional Formularies

Liquid Hope Adult Formula

Liquid Hope is the world's first shelf-stable organic whole foods meal replacement or supplement for oral and enteral use. It is formulated to help maintain healthy weight and support lean body tissue maintenance and repair.

"Functional formulas were created out of Love, Necessity and Hope for our founder's father who suffered a traumatic brain injury. After an extensive search to find a real, whole-foods feeding tube formula came up empty handed, our founder created one. Out of this passionate journey fueled by love and perseverance, came Liquid Hope, the world's first shelf-stable organic, whole-food feeding tube formula."

functionalformularies.com

Carewell: The Caregivers Shop

Compleat Organic Blends Enteral Feeding Tube Formula

carewell.com

Real Food Blends

Real food blends for feeding tubes that are covered by many insurance companies.

realfoodblends.com

Kate Farms

Offers a calorically dense, peptide-based nutritional formula made for sole-source or supplemental nutrition for drinking or tube feeding.

katefarms.com

Harvest

PediaSure Harvest and Ensure Harvest are made with pureed organic fruits and vegetables.

bringintheharvest.com

Other Feeding Tube Support

Feeding Tube and TPM Patients Zoom Support Group

For feeding tube and/or TPN patients and caregivers. For the Zoom link, email Hadar (address below). You will be added to the email list and receive a new Zoom link every month.

hadarbirger@hotmail.com

Blenderized RN

This page on Facebook is run by a registered nurse offering real blended food consulting for both children and adults with a g-tube. Discussions are only about real food and blending topics.

BlenderizedRN.com

crunchytubiemama.com

Matthews Manna

Blenderized wholefood recipes for individuals with gastric tubes and the entire family. Created by a mother whose son is disabled and has a g-tube. She shares what she has learned over the years.

matthewsmanna.com

Tubenmann Apparel

Tubenmann is the shirt that helps you dine out with dignity. Len Tubenmann designed a shirt that added a zipper to the mid area of the shirt so that you can easily and discreetly access your feeding tube. This re-opens the door to sitting down to meals and drinking with others without embarrassment.

facebook.com/tubenmannapparel

Dysphagia Cookbooks

Achilles, Elayne. **The Dysphagia Cookbook: Great Tasting and Nutritious Recipes for People with Swallowing Difficulties.** Cumberland House (2004). 9781581823486

Jeeris, Noah. **Dysphagia Cookbook Main Course.** Independently published (2019). Available on Amazon. 9781702810227

Woodruff, Sandra, and Gilbert-Henderson, Leah. **Soft Foods for Easier Eating Cookbook: Easy-to-Follow Recipes for People Who Have Chewing and Swallowing Problems.** Independently published (2009). ASIN B0157JH80S

Morris, Julie. **Superfood Smoothies – 110 Delicious, Energizing and Nutrient Dense Recipes.** Sterling; Illustrated edition (2013). 978-1454905592

Weihofen, Donna L. **Easy-to-Swallow, Easy-to-Chew Cookbook: Over 150 Tasty and Nutritious Recipes For People Who Have Difficulty Swallowing.** Houghton Mifflin (2002). ASIN B007SLV58U

Sayadi, Roya and Herskowitz, Joel. **Swallow Safely. How Swallowing Problems Threaten the Elderly and Others. A Caregiver's Guide to Recognition, Treatment and Prevention.** Inside/Outside Press (2010). ASIN *B00N4IJ2AE*

Freeman, Robert. **Easy Eating Cookbook: Tasty Recipes for Dysphagia and Hard to Swallow Conditions.** Independently published (2021). 9780645020908

Recipes on the Web

Wolff, Diane. *Essential Puree.*
Essential Puree is a site with ideas and books with pureed food recipes. It is a great help for those with dysphagia.
(essentialpuree.com).

Instructional videos for pureeing and dysphagia meals

Dysphagia-The Pureed Diet Made Easy
Foodservice Express
This video demonstrates the process of pureeing with tips for serving attractive pureed foods. It covers allowable foods as well as foods to avoid. It is very helpful with basic information for patients or caregivers.
youtube.com/watch?v=6urEz2ynTnk

Pureed Vegetable Recipe
Converse and Cook with Julie Effe
youtube.com/watch?v=4TWY1YQRwGQ

People With Swallowing Problems – Pureed food
North West Boroughs Healthcare
Video with dysphagia chefs Preston and James from Oak House Kitchen, in England. Here the chefs discuss how to modify a meal "to comply with international standards for people requiring a level 4 pureed diet."
youtube.com/watch?v=-va5tIDlPG0

How to Cook Delicious Pureed Meals for Seniors
Home Care Assistance
youtube.com/watch?v=QUTOY-MQzU0

Dysphagia Divas—Let's Puree!
Foodservice Express
"The Dysphagia Divas demonstrate how easy it is to puree almost

any food...even a tossed lettuce salad!" Other <u>Dysphagia Divas</u> videos, including for pureeing pizza and sandwiches, can be found on YouTube's Foodservice Express channel.

youtube.com/watch?v=SBOyO0WqiGo&t=2s

Breakfast Ideas for Parkinson Patient With Swallowing Disorder
Mary's Recipes
This video gives a clear, simple demo of how to make breakfast for those with dysphagia. There is no narration but the visual step-by-step how-to instruction is easy to follow.

youtube.com/watch?v=uiy9saRvpm8

No Chew Food for Soft Food & Puree Diets: Cheeseburgers
Sherri Smith
This unique video demonstrates how to puree a burger, and then mold it back into the shape of one. Be sure to browse Smith's "No Chew Food for Soft Food" series which present recipes with step-by-step visual instruction for cooking a variety of soft foods. You can adjust her recipes for your level of dysphagia.

youtube.com/watch?v=qFGGM9Z6b4w&t=47s

Most of the creators listed above have other relevant videos. You can easily locate their channels by filtering your YouTube search query by "channel." Also, if you search for the term "dysphagia recipe" in YouTube, you will find a trove of videos, too.

Nutritional Support for Dysphagia
From Those Who Have Experienced It Firsthand

"When my son was released from the hospital, we were released
with no aftercare plan in regards to nutrition. Basically, I was
like a deer in the headlights thinking, Oh crap! Now how do I feed
my son! I had no guidance on how to make his food. We had a
dietitian who was unwilling to share the blendable recipe she used
at the hospital. Finally, after weeks, she gave it to me. As if it this
was big secret she couldn't relinquish..."

—Jill (mother of a dysphagia patient)

I wrote earlier how in 1995 I was not sent to a swallow therapist, even after being diagnosed with severe dysphagia. I also had no nutritional help. This should never have been the case, but it was not unusual at that time. I wish there had been more support, so I did not have to figure everything out on my own.

Many years later, I did see a nutritionist. Unfortunately, my insurance did not cover it, but even having one session with her was helpful. If you are having trouble, ask your doctor or the hospital to send you to a nutritionist who can help you create a proper meal plan. If you do have a swallowing therapist, they will be able to refer you to someone who is a dietician or nutritionist, and that is what is supposed to be done. In talking to other dysphagia patients over the years and also taking a survey recently, it seems like half the people were sent to a dietician and half were not. I was shocked at the number of people who were not given nutritional help. I had assumed that perhaps I had just fallen through the cracks, but now I see there truly is not enough help for dysphagia patients. Many people fall through the cracks. The people who did get more help advocated for themselves and then were sent to a nutritionist through their swallowing therapist or doctor. Again, advocate for yourself or your loved one. That can make all the difference in getting the help you need.

Jill, the mother of a dysphagia patient quoted above, had to fight just to get the safe recipe from the dietician. Another woman told me after cancer surgery the doctor at the cancer center told her to feed him yogurt and Ensure drinks, but never once mentioned puree food or other options one can create in a blender. She did the research herself and found help through support groups. It was there that she was educated about how to create a healthy puree diet for her loved one. A fellow dysphagia patient named Glenn shared with me how his oncologist did send him to a nutritionist to help him with dysphagia. "It was a lifesaver," he wrote. He was lucky in that he had a doctor who understood the importance of referring patients to specialists who can help nutritionally.

The most important tip I can give you is to advocate for yourself just like Jill did for her son.

Just recently, a chef at a U.K. Care Center with a Dementia Unit joined a dysphagia recipe group looking for tips on what to make for the patients with swallow issues to gain weight. He saw that the food service they were using was not good enough and wanted to try a more natural approach. I gave him some of the tips I have mentioned in this book. It is a good thing that even Care Centers are beginning to understand the importance of a more natural approach to dysphagia instead of institutional unhealthy food. Food is medicine, and even with dysphagia, it is important to remember! With the right information and nutritional support, you can not only get enough calories, but you can also use healthy alternatives that will strengthen and heal the body. A nutritionist can also recommend what vitamins would be helpful for you or your loved one to add to their dysphagia diet.

When I did make an appointment with a holistic nutritionist, I made a point of asking her if she had worked with dysphagia patients. She had worked in a hospital for years and assured me she had worked with clients who had swallowing disorders. This made all the difference, and I felt very comfortable working with her. The experience was helpful and is something that should have been offered to me when I was diagnosed.

Nutritional Support Resources

Laura Michael
Nutritionist
Laura Michael is a nutritionist who works with people with swallowing disorders. She helps those living with dysphagia manage the changes in the textures of foods and beverages that they will need to thrive with the condition. Laura offers a comprehensive assessment of diet, eating pattern food preferences, both before and after the diagnosis, with the goal of getting someone as close as possible to the way they ate before dysphagia. She also teaches simple cooking methods and tips to adjust "regular" foods so eating (and cooking) can be pleasurable again.

Through her assessment and counseling, Laura can help someone make changes to their nutritional intake so they can be healthier and manage other disease conditions. Laura offers a 20-minute phone assessment at no cost. Should someone want to continue services, a zoom or phone meeting will be scheduled. Nutritional services start with a 5-day eating/diet assessment form for the client and for the caregiver to complete so Laura can get a snapshot of lifestyle and food preferences. Laura practices in Arizona (Mountain Standard Time).

Telephone: 480-266-5622.
Email: LEM.DSD@gmail.com

Niamh Condon

Dysphagia Nutritional Consultant

Niamh Condon is a chef with over 20 years' experience in the catering industry, and now over six years in the aged care sector. Niamh is a compassionate soul, who faced challenges morally about the standard way in which pureed food was cooked and presented to patients. It encouraged her to explore and innovate ways to give people pleasure from food again regardless of the swallowing. She can provide you with practical, simple, yet very effective methods of preparing meals for patients and caregivers. Simple tips, recipes and training are all available here. Based in Ireland, Niamh offers zoom or phone consults for patients, their caregivers and healthcare institutions throughout the world. For a consultation you can contact her through the contact form on the website listed above or find her on

diningwithdignity.ie

Instagram: *@dysphagiachef*

Diane Wolf

Diane Wolff has written the number one guidebook for setting up the dysphagia kitchen. She is author of *Seasons Of Puree Cookbooks*, using seasonal ingredients and cooking techniques for variety and healing. She is also the only independent publisher in the US who has created a library of books for patients with swallowing disorders.

Diane is available by personal appointment to do live cooking lecture demos. She does both live and virtual sessions. Diane also consults for a healthcare facility or a family healthcare situation. Fees depend on what is desired.

Visit her Instagram channel for recipes, tips and techniques.

@essentialpuree

Diane's YouTube channel, "Essential Puree: The Dysphagia Kitchen" has many cooking videos.

youtube.com/channel/UCTW9fQv5bzHv_E0G2pRPExA

Essential Puree is now in development for a frozen pureed food line. Those who are interested should write to Diane at:

diane@essentialpuree.com

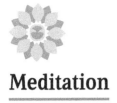

Meditation

"Resting is not laziness, it's medicine!"

—Glenn Schweitzer

Self-care is very important for everyone. It is a term that is thrown around a lot now but is more important than ever. Everyday life can be stressful, but dealing with a chronic illness and dysphagia is an added stress. For the last five years, I have practiced Transcendental Meditation (TM). It is a mantra-based meditation that is practiced two times a day. Live Zoom calls are now offered where thousands gather virtually to meditate together. I have found it very helpful. When I learned TM, I did get a discount due to my disability, and it was well worth it. It is a tool I now have for the rest of my life.

www.tm.org

There are many forms of meditation available for free as well. I have listed meditation apps below; some have a free trial period. Just sitting and taking deep breaths can help us. Grounding is a good technique too. As you sit and breathe, focus on your feet. I imagine roots coming out of my feet and going into the ground as if I am a tree. Most often, just putting my attention on the feet and breathing deeply is enough to ground me. I was taught this tool by an acupuncturist, and it helps me immediately. We are often so much in our heads and our worries that we forget that just sitting for a moment, breathing and grounding, can be all we need to get out of an anxious state. I also watch nature videos with music on YouTube and have found them very relaxing. There is one walk on the shores of Hawaii that is beautiful, and another is a walk down the Grand Canyon.

Getting the best nutrition along with calming techniques and practicing loving kindness toward ourselves, no matter what we are going through, is what self-care is all about. If you are a caregiver for someone with dysphagia, this is equally important for you too.

"Breathing techniques are so important for anyone with any kind of health condition, especially ones that increase stress levels . . . I pray as well as meditate and incorporate gratitude into both. It's not possible to feel overwhelmed or stressed while one is deeply immersed in gratitude." Jennie Hanning, Adv. Dip. and dysphagia patient

Meditation Apps

Headspace
headspace.com/headspace-meditation-app

Calm
calm.com

Portal: Escape Into Nature (for Mac).
"Portal transforms your surroundings and transports you to some of the most peaceful and awe-inspiring places on the planet, reconnecting you with nature."
portal.app

(Note: Some apps have free trial periods.)

Free Meditations

Jon Kabat Zinn
Jon Kabat-Zinn is an American professor emeritus of medicine and the creator of the Stress Reduction Clinic and the Center for Mindfulness in Medicine, Health Care, and Society at the University of Massachusetts Medical School. He is well respected, and his voice

is very calming. I highly recommend his meditations. You will find many free guided mindfulness meditations by Zinn, as well as lectures and interviews, available via different channels. Just search for him by name to see the offerings.

UCLA Health
Free guided meditations.
uclahealth.org/marc/mindful-meditations

3 Hour Crystal Singing Bowl Healing Sound Bath
Relaxing, meditative healing music. This video is very calming and beautiful. It has over four million views. I was told about this video by another dysphagia patient who recommended it, and now it is a resource I go to often. You can use it for meditation or simpy for relaxing healing music for your environment.
youtube.com/watch?v=gq8snFSEwlU&t=953s

Donna Eden Energy Medicine Kit
Sounds True
This is a ten-minute guided daily energy routine to strengthen and heal the body. I was reminded of it recently when an integrative doctor at Weill Cornell mentioned it to me to help heal while recovering from COVID. I did this simple ten-minute energy routine years ago and it was helpful and balancing.
youtube.com/watch?v=0nKWaJBgJ68

Marisa Peer—Healing Hypnosis
I have found Peer's "Do This To Completely HEAL Your Body and Mind" healing hypnosis video helpful, and recommend listening to this with regularity. You can find it on the "Mindvalley Talks" channel. URL is listed below, but you may find it easier to just search on YouTube by the video name.
www.youtube.com/channel/UCPvLJ7YsMqPWkHEfv4ftFZQ

Classes

There are also online classes to learn mindfulness meditation. It has been proven to help with stress and reduce pain levels. Mindfulness is often mentioned with those with dysphagia too to use when eating. When we are fully present, mindful, and calm, it is easier to eat in a safer manner.

With dysphagia, I have found that it is also best to eat in a quiet environment. I know this can often be difficult in certain circumstances, but because I have to focus on eating and swallowing, I have found that I do best being mindful and as relaxed as possible. This is where the practice of meditation becomes helpful in retraining the brain.

Benefits

A caregiver for a family member with dysphagia told me that meditation helps her keep her blood pressure down. A patient with dysphagia shared how both meditation and prayer helped them to deal with the physical and psychological aspects of this disorder. Another person mentioned gentle chair yoga. There are many things not in our control, and these are steps we can take to help our mental, physical, spiritual, and emotional health. Part of healing and being in our power is taking these steps and being kind to ourselves along the way.

Products

Capable Blankets
These are weighted blankets that are washable and help with anxiety and even PTSD. I tried using a weighted blanket years ago, but it was too heavy, which limited its use. Also it wasn't washable. A friend told me about Capable, and I have been very impressed. The blanket has helped with sleep and anxiety. It is even used in medical clinics while people are going through treatments. I also use it while doing

meditation, and it helps me feel protected and calm and allows for a deeper meditation. Because of Capable's SmartWeight technology, you never have to worry about setting a time limit on how long you use your blanket. All the Capable weighted products are designed to be safely used or worn without time constraints.

capeable.com

Complementary and Alternative Therapies

"Healing is akin to weeding and nourishing a garden, not solving a math problem."

—Abdi Assadi,
Acupuncturist and spiritual counselor

Because I was not offered any treatment or help through traditional medicine, I had to look for other forms of healing for help. My issue was neurological, so there was no surgery. I remember being given a medicine to help motility , but it did not do anything for me. I then turned to holistic doctors and practitioners, and I do believe that is what kept me alive. In the early days, I even got vitamin IVs from a holistic MD because I was so depleted from lack of food. What did help me were acupuncture, chiropractic, cranial sacral therapy, herbs, medical massage, and other natural treatments.

Research has shown how these alternative supportive therapies do help. Many major hospitals now have integrative medicine clinics. Memorial-Sloan Kettering Hospital has an Integrative Center only a few blocks from me, where acupuncture, cranial sacral therapy, medical massage, meditation, and nutritional support are offered to both inpatients and outpatients. New York-Presbyterian and Weill Cornell Medicine has also recently opened an Integrative Health and Wellbeing Center.

"Several academic medical centers across the country are starting to offer these services, and patients are benefiting tremendously," says Dr. Chiti Parikh, noting that there is considerable research that supports the use of integrative methods. "As one of the top

healthcare institutions in the country, we knew we had to offer
these services to our patients and employees."
—Weill-Cornell "Newsroom"
news.weill.cornell.edu/news/2017/12/
is-integrative-health-the-future-of-medicine

Jon Kabat-Zinn, on the faculty of the University of Massachusetts Medical School, founded the Stress Reduction Clinic to teach mindfulness-based techniques and mindfulness meditation. This was back in 1979 when it was revolutionary to do so. He created a secularized eight-week mindfulness course called Mindfulness-Based Stress Reduction (MBSR) to help patients with chronic pain and stress. It has helped many people with illness, as much of illness is made worse or worsened by stress. The joining of Eastern practices and meditation in hospitals now just shows how traditional and holistic alternative medicine practices go hand in hand in the healing process. I took the MBSR course at Sloan Kettering Hospital seven years ago and found it very helpful.

During many years of dealing with chronic illness and dysphagia, I found some very good practitioners who I believe saved my life. If you do not live near an integrative center associated with a hospital, I would suggest referrals or word of mouth. One of the best chiropractors I have found does not advertise, and all his patients are from word of mouth. Be discerning and do research just as you would when going to any doctor. Recently, a newly diagnosed dysphagia patient told me a chiropractor helped her in a very short time. Make sure the practitioner is certified. Often these alternative therapies can be helpful and complementary to any traditional treatment you are receiving. I have heard from other dysphagia patients how acupuncture was helpful too. It is another resource that is now available and more widely accepted than years ago.

Emotional Support

"Sometimes you will be in control of your illness and other times you'll sink into despair, and that's OK! Freak out, forgive yourself, and try again tomorrow."

—Kelly Hemingway

"Our society revolves around food and meals. For people with dysphagia, life as you know it ceases to exist. Dysphagia can cause depression, low self-esteem, lost wages, poor social performance, and increasing health risks such as aspiration pneumonia. Working through the mental aspects of this disorder is, in many ways, as challenging as addressing the physical limitations."

—National Foundation of Swallowing Disorders (NFOSD)
swallowingdisorderfoundation.com

For years, I did not have any form of counseling, as I was unable to find a good therapist. I know from talking to others this is not uncommon. Either the therapists did not take my insurance, or they did not understand the complexities of living with a disability or chronic illness. I once went to a social worker who just assumed dysphagia was a mental issue because she had never heard of it. When she told me that, I never returned. Even before I had a swallowing disorder, I knew people in the world were on feeding tubes and had swallowing issues due to various disabilities.

When I went to a well-known hospital swallowing center for treatment, I asked for a therapist to help me with all the loss and change of life that comes with dysphagia. The head of the department told me they only had psychologists for their patients with swallowing phobias. I stood there shocked. That they did not even think the patients who can no longer eat normally did not need psychological help still astounds me to this day. I hope things will start to change in this area and the proper help is given and more understanding is shown.

There are good therapists out there, though. Make sure they understand chronic illness. When I asked a psychologist who specializes in helping those with chronic illness and brain injury what was the most important advice I could give, her response was to make sure the therapist has an understanding of working with people with disabilities. Specifically, she emphasized that specialists called rehabilitation psychologists work with people with disabilities and chronic disabling illness. (abpp.org/Directory)

I have listed the National Foundation of Swallowing Disorders above, and they may have names of people who offer emotional help. They also offer virtual support groups, which might be of help to you or your loved one. If you need to talk to a counselor, you can also look for help through a spiritual advisor from your church, temple, or other houses of worship.

I have heard people in dysphagia support groups express how painful it is to be around others eating. I know that feeling. It was so uncomfortable for me and brought up so much grief and anger that I began to avoid it at all costs. But doing so only made me feel lonelier and sadder. Having dysphagia is very isolating and can also be painful for the family to eat around the patient. There is much loss and grief that is part of living with dysphagia, and that is why it is important to have some form of support. I do know if I had support earlier on, it would have been very helpful. I do agree with the quote above from the swallowing foundation website. The psychological effects of dysphagia were just as difficult if not more so than the physical. It affected every area of my life. Again, this is why it is so important to have some form of emotional and/or spiritual help during this time.

Rehabilitation centers have rehabilitation psychologists. These psychologists are trained to work with patients with severe disabilities and so would understand dysphagia. Ask at your hospital or rehab center if there is a rehab psychologist who can work with you. The therapist who finally was able to help me is a rehab psychologist who has an outpatient practice. There are other therapists who do work with people with illness and disability other than rehab psychologists. It may take time to build a team with support that works for you. Advocate for yourself, and do not give up. Before I found a therapist who was good and able to help me with the years of accumulated trauma from all of this, I had given up. I was even told by others not to even look anymore and that it was hopeless. If I had listened to them, I would never have gotten the help I so deserved. Again, advocate for yourself or your loved one. It can take time and effort, but help is there.

Psychology Today

You can look for therapists through the *Psychology Today* website. You are able to filter through what insurance you have and what kind of therapy you are looking for.

www.psychologytoday.com/us

BetterHelp

Online therapy tailored to your needs. BetterHelp offers access to licensed, trained, experienced, and accredited psychologists (PhD/PsyD), marriage and family therapists (LMFT), clinical social workers (LCSW / LMSW), and board licensed professional counselors (LPC).

www.betterhelp.com

"This is a moment of suffering. Suffering is part of life. May I be kind to myself in this moment. May I give myself the compassion I need."

—Kristen Neff

Support groups and Foundations

National Foundation of Swallowing Disorders (NFOSD)

NFOSD is a wonderful foundation for helping those with swallowing disorders. Their commitment is to provide patients hope and improve the quality of life for those with swallowing disorders.

NFOSD offers Zoom virtual support calls once a month for those with dysphagia and another one for caregivers. I was on the latest Zoom group call, and it was a very emotional experience for me. It was the first time in all the years I have had dysphagia that I was in a support group atmosphere. The experience of support from others in the group is very healing. We shared our stories and our concerns. We shared our hopes and what we wish we had known. Every person in the group seemed so grateful because nobody else can understand what it is like to live with dysphagia. To have the support of others who do understand is a blessing. NFOSD also has a support group for parents of children with swallowing disorders and one for caregivers. Look on the site for more information. This foundation offers the most help and information available on the Internet that I have found to date.

swallowingdisorderfoundation.com

International Dysphagia Diet Standardization Initiative

"The IDDSI committee came together in 2013 with the goal of developing international standardized terminology and descriptors for dysphagia diets that would meet the needs of individuals with dysphagia across the age span, across all care setting and across all cultures." From the IDDSI site, many resources and food charts on the site.

(IDDSI) iddsi.org

Beyond My Battle

A site dedicated to reducing the stress of serious illness, rare disease, and disability through emotional support and educational resources rooted in mindfulness, awareness, and compassion. They also offer Zoom support groups for both patients and caregivers.

beyondmybattle.org

Oakhouse Kitchen

This site has many helpful links and resources for those with dysphagia. They have a recipes for dysphagia hub on this site, including a dysphagia recipe of the month section.

oakhouse-kitchen.com

Facebook Support Groups

The groups and pages listed below offer mutual peer support and are invaluable.

- NFOSD Online Swallowing Support Group
  groups/NFOSDSwallowingSupportGroup

- National Foundation of Swallowing Disorders
  facebook.com/nfosd

- Dysphagia food & recipes group
  facebook.com/groups/271415403304438

- Dysphagia/swallowing support group
  facebook.com/groups/450737689527997

- Dysphagia café
  facebook.com/dysphagiacafe

- Esophageal Dysmotility Disorder group
  facebook.com/groups/1064795553610874

- Blenderized RN
  facebook.com/groups/BlenderizedRN

- Cake Method (Dysphagia - Puree & Soft Food Diets)
  facebook.com/groups/cakemethod

  Created by a caregiver who cooks for a patient with dysphagia.

- Caring for the Caregiver Support Group
  facebook.com/groups/1491221791165989

  Support for all caregivers.

" Go Back and take care of yourself. Your body needs you, your feelings need you, your perceptions need you. Your suffering needs you to acknowledge it. Go home and be there for all these things."

—Thich Nhat Hanh

Supportive Books and Videos

My Three Belly Buttons by John Bruce. Lulu.com (2011). 9781105169793.
An open, frank narrative of one man's emotional battle with cancer, starting with diagnosis, dealing with the surgery, dysphagia, and treatments that followed. I highly recommend John's book if you too are dealing with dysphagia due to cancer and cancer treatments.

Chödrön, Pema. **When Things Fall Apart: Heart Advice for Difficult Times.** Shambhala (2016). 9781611803433

Bernhard, Toni. **How to Live Well with Chronic Pain and Illness: A Mindful Guide.** Wisdom Publications (2015). 9781614292487
For patients and their caregivers.

Kate Lorig, RN, Dr. Phd; Holman, Halsted, MD; Sobel, David, MD, MPH; Laurent, Diania, MPH; Gonzalez, Virginia, MPH; and Minor, Marion, RPT, PhD. **Living a Healthy Life with Chronic Conditions.** Bull Publishing Company; Fifth edition (2020). 9781945188312

Kabat-Zinn, Jon. **Full Catastrophe Living: Using the Wisdom of Your Body and Mind to Face Stress, Pain, and Illness.** Bantam; Revised edition (2013). 9780345536938

Ruiz, Don Miguel. **The Four Agreements: A Practical Guide to Personal Freedom (A Toltec Wisdom Book).** Amber-Allen Publishing (2018). 9781878424310
The Four Agreements reveals the source of self-limiting beliefs that rob us of joy and create needless suffering.

Scher, Amy B. **How to Heal Yourself When No One Else Can: A Total Self-Healing Approach for Mind, Body, and Spirit.** Llewellyn

Publications (2016). 9780738745541

Brach, Tara. **Radical Compassion: Learning to Love Yourself and Your World with the Practice of RAIN.** Penguin Life (2019). 9780525522812

Frankl, Viktor E. **Man's Search for Meaning.** Beacon Press; Gift edition (2014, originally published in 1946). 9780323306577. (*Other editions available in stores and online.*)
One cognitive psychologist informed me that she recommends *Man's Search for Meaning to* patients who are living with severe illness or disability and/or are going through life changes. I read it years ago and it has always been one of my favorite books. It teaches about the importance of purpose even in the most horrifying circumstances.

Cousins, Norman. **Anatomy of an Illness as Perceived by the Patient: Reflections on Healing and Regeneration.** W. W. Norton & Company (2001, originally published in 1979). 9780393041903

Jackson, Suzan. **Finding a New Normal: Living Your Best Life with Chronic Illness.** Independently published (2020). 9781734299014

Hanning, Jennifer. **Stepping Stones to Meditation.** Independently published (2013). 9781483959016
Written by a dysphagia patient who is also a meditation teacher.

Lake, Doug, MD., **Esophagus Attack!: The 3-Step Method to Enjoy Eating Again.** Lioncrest Publishing (2021). 9781544516974
For patients with swallowing issues related to Gastroesophageal Reflux disease (GERD). The book also offers support for patients who get food caught in their esophagus.

Sayadi, Roya and Herskowitz, Joel. **Swallow Safely. How Swallowing Problems Threaten the Elderly and Others.** (See page 36)

Loyd, Rita. **Unconditional Self-Love.** Nurturing Art Publishing (2010). 9780615378879. *2nd Edition* can be purchased directly through the author's web site: *nuturingart.com*

Documentaries and YouTube Ted Talks

Swallow: A Documentary—Dysphagia.
Can be found on YouTube and the NFOSD website.

swallowingdisorderfoundation.com/swallow-a-documentary

Unable To Swallow- A Patient's Story of Years of Living with Achalasia.
Chris suffered for years with Achalasia, a disease that prevented him from swallowing food or even water. A hopeful story of a new medical procedure that helped him.

columbiasurgery.org/stories/unable-swallow-patients-story-years-living-achalasia

Confronting Chronic Disease and Refusing To Give Up
Susannah Meadows | TEDxNashville.

In this moving, personal talk, Susannah Meadows shares what she learned about hope and the refusal to give up. She also delves into the science to show why perseverance itself may be a prescription for recovery. A talk about thinking outside the box in healing and the importance of perseverance.

.youtube.com/watch?v=L9fjn3PqOXI

My Philosophy for a Happy Life
Sam Berns | TEDxMidAtlantic

The speaker, Sam Berns, had Progeria. His talk about his simple philosophy for having a happy life no matter what challenges we face is beautiful. His legacy lives on and his wisdom still helps others.

ted.com/talks/sam_berns_my_philosophy_for_a_happy_life?language=en

The Prison of Your Mind
Sean Stephenson-Tedx

Sean Clinch Stephenson was an American therapist, self-help author and motivational speaker. Because he was born with osteogenesis imperfecta, Stephenson stood three feet tall, had fragile bones, and used a wheelchair. This talk on You Tube is inspiring and teaches about the importance of self love and the prison of the mind.

youtube.com/watch?v=VaRO5-V1uK0

Laughter as Medicine and Self-Care

"Laughter is a powerful way to tap positive emotions."

—Dr. Norman Cousins

Years ago, I read a book by Dr. Norman Cousins called *Anatomy of an Illness.* Dr. Cousins suffered from an incurable illness and used what he called "laughter therapy" to heal. His studies of how laughter and positive thinking helped people heal helped inspire the holistic health movement. "We mustn't regard any of this as a substitute for competent medical attention," he said in an interview. "But the doctor can only do half the job. The other half is the patient's response to the illness." That is true.

I have found laughter to be extraordinarily healing. When I laugh out loud—a real laugh—I feel alive. I feel there is hope. I can feel my mood changes as well as my outlook. My father used to say, "Where there is life there is hope." I will add to that and say, "Where there is laughter there is hope." Mel Brooks talks about how he survived serving during WW2 by using humor. That was his way of dealing with the horrors around him, and of course he later made some of the funniest movies ever made.

Part of self-care can be watching funny shows or listening to humorous podcasts or radio shows. I turn to clips of Don Rickles or other comedians on YouTube. I also listen to a well-known radio comedy show at times. It was this show through the years that often got me through hard times because I always laughed at the sarcastic humor. My mother once told me that she heard me laughing while listening to the show, and she knew I was going to be okay. She repeated that story often, so it must have given her hope to hear me laugh when she saw that I was having such difficult times. Dr. Norman Cousins watched the Marx Brothers and Candid Camera, as they both made him laugh. Find what makes you laugh and laugh.

I believe humor has helped me survive all I have been through, and this is why I decided to add this section to this book. I notice that when things are worse, I am more sarcastic and funnier. It has been a coping mechanism for me as it is for many others. Many scientific studies have been done on the health benefits of laughter and smiling, and you can find many of these articles and studies on the internet if you would like to learn more about this. I know laughter is healing. I have never known anyone who said they feel worse when they are laughing, and I have always felt better when I laugh.

I started watching the Marx Brothers' movies while writing this book. Although I knew who Groucho was, I had never watched any of the Marx Brothers' movies in full before. Not only did I find them funny but healing as well. There is a certain rhythm and energy to them that was relaxing too. I also began to watch You Bet Your Life episodes on YouTube starring Groucho Marx. I laughed out loud many times at a game show that was filmed more than ten years before I was even born. I have watched so many old clips of Groucho in the last month that I sometimes hear his jokes in my head. Of course, I hear them in his voice. If I start smoking a cigar and making witty putdown comments to people on my block, then I will know I have watched one too many of his clips and will stop. But for now, I think I am okay. I do now understand why Dr. Norman Cousins watched so many Marx Brothers' movies when he was so ill.

Years ago, I attended a mindfulness meditation class. The teacher talked about the importance of smiling and how a simple smile can trick the brain into thinking we are happy and shift our mood. The teacher told us that even just smiling tricks the brain into thinking we are happy and is healing. I do this even at my lowest, and I can feel it change me—just the act of smiling even when I do not feel like it often can get me out of very negative thinking and lower moods. I can notice the change. Try it.

Again, the reason I focus on laughter in this resource book is because I know firsthand how difficult living with dysphagia is. I understand, and there have been many times dealing with it and illness that I wanted to give up. I know from talking to other patients they too have dealt with dark nights of the soul like I have. I say hold on. Do the best you can. Take it one moment at a time, and laugh. And as Groucho said, "If you find it hard to laugh at yourself, I would be happy to do it for you."

"In the moment of a laugh, you forget
every problem you've ever had."

—*Jerry Seinfeld*

Self-Care as Nourishment
and Other Gentle Reminders

"There is enough guilt in the world. There are enough shoulds in the world. Be gentle with yourself."

—Bob Roth,

American Transcendental Meditation teacher and author.

Nourishment is a core issue when one has dysphagia, but there are many forms of nourishment. Nourishment is not just food. Self-care is nourishment too. Being kind to yourself is nourishment. It is easy to forget to self-nourish. Make sure to rest when you need it—allow yourself to grieve and feel your feelings. Allow yourself to feel them, but also know when you need to distract yourself so you do not drown in it. Forms of distraction could be watching a funny movie, reading an uplifting book, or calling a friend. If you find that you are "alone" and feel no support, this is the time to be the support you need.

A wise woman recently told me to not go to an empty well for a drink of water. She was talking about expecting compassion and help from those who are incapable of showing up for us and never have. I had done this a lot in my life, as we often do. The energy and anger wasted is energy, and our energy is precious. We are precious. I bring this up because many people with chronic illness and especially invisible illnesses have much trauma around people not understanding or not being there for them. Again, do not go to an empty well for water. We are the ones who are responsible for showing up for ourselves, and that is what we can control. The ultimate form of self-nourishment is self-love.

We often do not even know how to nourish ourselves. We are not really taught it. We often hear the negative voices of others or ourselves far louder than the kind ones, and so it is a relearning. Begin to notice your thoughts. When you hear yourself tell yourself an untruth or an unkind word, stop and replace it with kindness. Stop and be kind to yourself now. When I find myself being hard on myself, I will stop and think of all I have been through and wonder if I would talk like that to someone else going through this. If the answer is no, then I remind myself to be kind to myself instead.

For myself, I have always been an over doer—always trying to figure out things. I believe it is from so many years of having to figure out how to survive an incredibly difficult and unknown illness and, so it is now automatic for me but can be so automatic that it is unhealthy. It can be exhausting. My neurologist is also one of the official doctors at mixed martial arts (MMA) fights. He once told me I am like a fighter in a ring who hears the bell to stop but does not stop. I related to that analogy so strongly and only later found out that he often had to stop the fights in real boxing rings when it was becoming too dangerous for one of the fighters. He would know and he was spot on with seeing that about me. A close friend of mine who knows this about me too sent me a quote years ago and told me to put it up where I could see it. I did put it up near my bed and often just seeing it helps shift that exhausting self. The quote is below:

"Let go of what has passed. Let go of what may come. Let go of what's happening now. Don't try to figure anything out. Don't try to make anything happen. Relax right now and rest." Tilopa

Look through pictures or quotes that might inspire you or create a shift for you as the one above does for me. I also bought a stuffed animal sloth and put it on a shelf to remind me to slow down. Sloths are very slow creatures. Look for quotes or pictures that are uplifting to you and hang it where you can see it as a reminder for you to be kind to yourself or to not give up. Maybe you are someone who needs to take more action or steps. Find quotes or mementos that remind you to take action or find something that gives you hope and faith. There are many companies on Etsy that will make a quote into a beautifully designed digital file that you can print out. I did that and framed it. The serenity prayer is another reminder I have hanging on the wall. "God, grant me the serenity to accept the things I cannot change, courage to change the things I can, and wisdom to know the difference" (Reinhold Niebuhr). This is a prayer that is often quoted and used in many 12-step programs.

There are days when self-care consists of me telling myself, "Just get through the day. You can do it." There have been many days when that was all I could muster to survive. I know many of you reading this can relate to this. Make a list of ways in which you have been hard on yourself or unkind words you tell yourself and another list of ways you can practice self-care and be kind to yourself instead. If you look at that list, you will get a better idea of things you might need to shift in order to be kinder to yourself and forms of self-care that would be beneficial to you. Sometimes we don't even realize how we are hard on ourselves or unkind—or even what we can do to nourish ourselves. How many times are we outraged by unkind words another says to us, and yet we abuse ourselves with unkind words every day?

One of the words of advice my father gave me was "You need to be your own best friend, Julia." He was right. He knew how hard I was on myself. Be your own ally and best friend. Be your own cheerleader when needed and nourish yourself the best you can. We don't have control over how others treat us or even if they will show up for us, but we do have control over how we treat ourselves. We do not have control over having dysphagia, but we can be in acceptance in the moment and be kind to ourselves while going through it. We can do all it takes to nourish ourselves now in all ways.

It is easy to focus on what we do not have and the people who are not there for us. That is the first place we go, of course. We are often conditioned to focus on what is lacking. Instead, focus on what you can control and let go as much as you can of what you cannot control. This is where the serenity prayer comes in as a reminder, which I listed above. This is the path of healing. One step at a time. One moment at a time. Be gentle with yourself. Do not give up or give up on yourself. Let the rest go. I know that as simple as this sounds, it is often the hardest thing we can do . . . and so I say again, it is a relearning. Relearning to release all the negative self-talk and storytelling we believe is true and have told ourselves forever is often not an easy task. I will find myself slipping into it, and I will then say gentle words to myself and remember to endorse all I have done and have been through. I put myself in the place of "My own best friend"— instead of my own worst enemy. Again, it is a relearning. It is not easy, especially when we are exhausted and so angry at the situation, but it is worth it and is part of the healing process, if you allow it. I see it as a gentle navigation change. When I start to go off course into self-defeating behavior or being too hard on myself, I redirect my direction toward self-compassion and send gentle words toward myself.

Today I was talking to my friend Rita Loyd. I have a lot on my plate (dysphagia pun intended), and she knew it was overwhelming for me. At the end of our talk, she said, "Do something that feeds your soul today, Julia. Do something that feeds your soul." It hit home. I smiled, thinking how that was what I wanted to convey in this book and this chapter. I also smiled because it was what I too so needed to hear today.

I had an appointment with a doctor after our talk, and on the way there I stopped at 179 E 93rd street. The building was only a few blocks from my doctor, and I had promised myself the next time I saw him I would go there. 179 E 93rd street is the childhood home of the Marx Brothers. I sat on the stoop for about an hour and just rested. I thought of how the street must have looked then and how the Marx Brothers played in these streets and ran up the stoop. My mind went to another time far away and long ago and visions of kids playing stickball in the street and early 1900s cars lining the block. I thought of how comedy genius came from the humble beginnings of a tenement building in old New York, and how incredible that is. A man stopped to take a photo, and I asked him if I should move out of the way. I thought he was taking it because of the history of the building. He was not. He said he was from the building department, and they were thinking of changing the building's façade, and so he was taking pictures. I told him that Groucho Marx had lived there in the early 1900s, and he said he had no idea. I then told him that Groucho Marx and I had the same birthday, October 2nd, but I added, "Not the same year. Groucho was born in 1890, and if I was born that year we would either have a big problem here or I look very, very, very good for my age." He laughed. I did not even find it a particularly funny joke, but he laughed. If I laugh, it feeds my soul, and if I make others laugh, it feeds my soul.

It is no surprise that my friend Rita teaches about self-compassion and is an artist whose work is based on unconditional self-love. Her words were just what I needed to hear. Be gentle with yourself. Be compassionate to yourself through this. As you learn to navigate the difficult task of nourishing yourself while having dysphagia, please do not forget to "feed your soul." What would feed your soul today? What can you do to feed your soul?

> *"If your compassion does not include*
> *yourself, it is incomplete."*
> —Jack Kornfield

Advice From Other Patients and caregivers

"Out of suffering have emerged the strongest souls; the most massive characters are seared with scars."

—Kahlil Gibran

The best advice comes from the people who have lived it. These brave souls all have dysphagia and agreed to give some advice that has helped them through their own swallowing issues. I am grateful for them agreeing to share their wisdom for this resource guide.

"My husband's dysphagia makes eating slow and a concentrated effort for him. He cannot also talk. So we look forward to watching an episode of a chosen TV series to keep us quiet and give us an hour to slowly eat."

—Julia Herron Ousley

"Use a small cup so too much can't slosh into your mouth."

—Nicola Black

"Learn relaxation techniques and mindfully relax the throat and chest area before each swallow."

—Jennie Hanning

"I cook for my husband who has PPA . It was trial and error but I have found that he can basically eat most things if you puree them and add liquid (chicken broth, beef broth depending on the food) until it gets to the consistency you can manage. I even took a piece of Chicago deep-dish pizza with sausage and pureed it with chicken broth. He loved it. For veggies, just get any bag of frozen, don't add water but cook on stove and when they are done, add 3 wedges of laughing cow cheese and then puree. Get real creamy and tasty with the laughing cow. Lost 17 lbs. before I figured this out and now has gained 13 back."

—Beth D.

"Get a thermos to put a heated-up pureed meal, a bowl, spoon, and place all in a nice cooler. Bring this to a restaurant. Pour the contents in a bowl to eat when the other guests have been served their meals. I use a thermos, which will keep food hot for five hours or more. Order a drink from the restaurant and a pudding-like dessert. Enjoy time out with the family or friends. When I do this, I feel as if I am not missing out on the social experience I so enjoy."

—Karen Griffey

"Hypnotherapy helped me immensely as I used it to relax before a meal."

—Janine

"The thing about dysphagia is the bullying you get from family and friends with the best of intentions and love; it's the 'you need more to eat than that' or that 'you have not put enough food on your plate' and then having to explain gets me down. I tell them

69

that I eat many times during the day, small amounts, which works for me. I also realize it is because of their love for me and concern, and I remind myself of that."

—Liz

"Acupuncture has been helping me throughout my diagnosis with dysphagia. I've had success with relieving pain and with assistance with relaxation. I highly recommend acupuncture for this issue, and for overall health is a holistic approach. Massage and chiropractic assistance has helped me as well, especially as he works on my vagus nerve."

—Lisa Duff Craft

"It can be a bit of a lonely road dealing with dysphagia whatever level (I have a feeding tube & puree), so reach out to support groups like this one. Help family and friends to understand and try to put them at ease about eating normally around you, as hard as that is, because they feel horrible too. I've also learned what may work for one may not be right for you. You are the one who has to work out what is right for you; it is your body. Also, flavor is very important, also lots of sauces, dressings, gravies, seasonings are the best when all else fails. You will have good days and bad, but don't give up. Also, try to find joy in other activities that don't always involve food. Explore new hobbies, enjoy nature, etc."

—Teena Thompson

"I don't have the condition, but work in social care with residents that are affected. I think that if I were to give any advice at all it would be to first learn about the patient in detail, I have found

this helps greatly with understanding how to prepare meals that maintain dignity in dining. I do believe that care needs to be taken to ingredient selection to ensure balanced nutrition and flavor. Some ingredients do not blend well. For example, the husks of garden peas can leave the food gritty. This would need to be blended to thin liquid, and pushed through a sieve and thickened up to the appropriate level on the IDDSI scale. Meats should be good quality cuts that are cooked tender and the outer edges removed. Adding meat stock instead of water to meat is helpful and more flavorful. Buy a powerful commercial stick blender and not a jug type blender.

For calorie intake I have a mini milkshake I make for patients which is around 500 kcal for 200ml. It is very easy and quick to make. I use 100ml double cream, a scoop of ice cream and a teaspoon of Nestle Nesquik flavoring. Blend and serve. It can be thickened up to the appropriate level before serving. The thickeners used with foods should be gum based and not starch based. Starch based thickener mixed with the Amylase in saliva thins the food, causing a potential choking hazard.

Also, the all important spoon test for level 4 is very helpful and simple test that ensures safety. You can look up what the spoon tilt test is for dysphagia online. I am now in the middle of a project to deliver level 4 meals to 4 care homes in my job and I am learning a lot. I also think that much like cooking and experimenting with regular food dishes, the same is applied to getting it right for dysphagia dishes. It is trial and error process. Repetition is the mother of learning. Keep trying."

—Andrew Brownridge

"I had throat cancer and the radiotherapy caused my dysphagia. Feeling grateful to still be here is what keeps me going! Tube fed 27 months now, but there are people with worse things." Sharon P.

"Most people don't ever think about it unless it happens to them or someone they know, and even then they rarely understand the psychological effects. I think the medical community often deems it as manageable, even if that's via not being able to swallow anymore at all, so there isn't enough done to address it or spread awareness. I am blessed in that I got into a good ENT (ear, nose, and throat) and a wonderful swallowing therapist, and I have a mental health counselor who also helps process the trauma. It's really awful to me to see that my experience isn't the standard. It makes me so sad to see how many people struggle to get care. Advocate for yourself as much as you can."

—Melissa

"Texture was everything for me. Smooth and silky/velvety to help it glide down. I used homemade cashew nut cream to add to the soups/smoothies, which also added extra, much-needed protein. Also coconut milk helps me get nutrition in the shakes and in soups. It was important to get as many calories in as possible as amounts became so limited."

—Cara

"I call all my dysphagia folks my family. I always try to remind them that we are eating to live and not living to eat. Invest in a good food processor/blender. I have three different blenders. One is a portable and it makes traveling possible. As I like to say, 'Have blender will travel.' There will be good and bad eating days but you can do it! On the bad days, push through to the better days."

—Felicia Thompson-Williams

"Practice mindful eating. During the meal, I am very focused on eating. I take each step—chewing, swallowing—slowly. I don't rush or try to eat foods I've had trouble with before, such as raw vegetables, rice, and dishes with whole nuts or pieces of them. I take a small bite of food, then chew and swallow it. I don't take another bite until I've completely swallowed the previous one."

—Leslie Krongold, EdD, *glasshalffull.online*

"I am a thirteen-year survivor of stage IV Squamous Cell Carcinoma of the head and neck region. My main treatment consisted of a radical neck dissection with forearm flap surgery, 30 doses of radiation, and a full regime of Cisplatin. The result of these treatments was that my anatomy for swallowing, general feeling or sensation in the mouth, and chewing were all adversely affected. Much of my saliva glands were completely destroyed or negatively affected by the treatment. Eating for me went from a what's on the menu today, to a cognitive analytical process and problem-solving exercise of what can I eat on this menu with the least amount of effort and how will it affect the social setting I am in, whether I be alone or with company. The reality of many head and neck cancer patients is that they have to start at the pureed everything food stage and through extreme concentration and hard work, improve their technique in eating to move toward some semblance of normalcy in food mitigating the effects of dysphagia related to the destruction of their saliva glands.

"Within the last 13 years I have developed an almost unconscious ability for chewing and swallowing some foods, that is the main challenge of dysphagia. With dysphagia you have to be constantly aware of every bite. Swallowing is a process that we as humans do continuously through life and take for granted until something goes wrong. Dysphagia complicates this process and brings swallowing to a conscious level, because if we forget what we are doing while

swallowing, the consequence could be choking and aspiration of food into our lungs, leading to all sorts of health challenges. Through hours of practice, I just know and have confidence that the problem of choking is negligible with a few easy foods, such as a banana. I don't have this freedom with the majority of foods, but as time goes by, my list of 'easy swallow food' grows and many do get easier. Portable tools that assist people with dysphagia are currently being developed to support people with dysphagia conditions at home, resulting in improved quality of life. This will become more important, as more people become survivors, and it will allow them to feel more comfortable with food in social settings. This action alone will alleviate many mental stress issues such as depression, isolation, and anxiety for these individuals, as it has me.

"I was also so focused on the physical part of healing, not realizing that I was pushing down the emotional trauma. Even when we try to avoid it, it will come up anyway, and we have to deal with the emotional and mental aspects to heal as well. The mental state is a fragile thing and food is such a social center and part of our culture and well-being. Healing is not just about the physical but also addressing the emotional aspect of this as well while going through it all. I wrote my book to heal myself and in turn, it has helped others going through a similar situation. For that I am grateful."

—John Bruce
Cancer survivor and author of *My Three Belly Buttons*

"It's been very hard to deal with, but acceptance has helped me. I tell myself things are not like they used to be and that can change too. There is something about self-talk and acceptance that has helped me deal with this loss. I try to focus on other things that are enjoyable for me that are not about food. I would tell others to accept where you are now and the situation. I do not know how to *tell people how to get there, but it has helped me to focus on what I can do."*

—Jen

"I have found much helpful information here and appreciate the recipes , ideas and support in dealing with my husband's difficult diet. It's critical that we feed him correctly as he ended up very, very ill from aspiration pneumonia in both lungs. We are hoping to avoid a feeding tube. My advice would be to experiment! So far, we have realized starches are tough for him; pasta, potatoes (other than mashed), and rice all turn rather glutinous and pasty when pureed and he doesn't have saliva either (from radiation). But the other day, I was looking for a starch/something to go with a creamy soup (pureed bacon lentil soup), so I took a couple of rusks (Swedish toasts) and poured warm broth over them. They kind of dissolve, but gave my husband the sensation of having something crunchy. I also highly recommend a segmented dish; more like eating a regular dinner but without needing a bunch of bowls to keep from running together. I got one on Amazon. Hope this is helpful."

Diane Martin

"In the beginning of my 'journey' I lost a lot of weight, and I'm already quite tiny, so that was the worst part for me. Now I'm a very healthy weight. Start counting calories to learn how to eat calorie-dense, healthy foods. MyFitnessPal is really good and simple to use. My main go-to smoothie is almond milk, dates, banana, peanut butter with some cocoa powder, and flax seeds. If you do one of these, plus a coconut milk and fruit smoothie later, that's almost everything you need. Avocado, eggs, bananas, butter, cheese, milk, coconut milk, beans, lentils—these are all

calorie-dense foods. I like to eat cheese with bone broth for a savory meal/snack."

Misty Lambert

"My diet is pureed and my advice is—focus on flavors! Close your eyes and try to taste all those yummy ingredients. Use the flavors you love, experiment and create new dishes for yourself. Just because it's pureed doesn't mean it has to be boring. If you find something you love, restrict how much you have a week so you don't get bored of it too quickly."

Ellie Morrish

"Find what works for you! Acupuncture, chiropractor, massage & Meditation helps me! Find doctors who support your journey. Invest in a food processor; I use a Vitamix & Magic Bullet Blender. Research supplements, vitamins and herbs to support your health. I utilize a nutritionist, too. Keep hope alive with a group like this on Facebook, support from family & friends. I have returned to therapy. Also, change your focus, or surrender and feel it all; it will pass. I have been making it a priority to do something I love every day!"

Lisa Helen

"Join the online dysphagia support groups. They have been a lifeline for me. The members 'live in your shoes' and understand how your every day is and feels. I also wish I knew that when you put too many vegetables in a soup and puree it, the end result would taste awful. I learned to use flavored balsamic blends, sauces, and spices. It was more flavorful if I cooked, seasoned, and pureed one food at a time and then put it on a plate. I enjoy the

experience of eating so much better. Take the time to batch cook and use silicone molds for food storage. Grab one serving and microwave when you are limited for time to cook. When going out, heat up your food, put it in a thermos, bring a bowl, spoon, and place them in a decorative cooler when going out for dinner."

—Karen Griffey

"An operation to remove a carotid body tumor in my neck in 2011 left my life changed immeasurably. I could never have imagined waking up with the total inability to swallow, not even my own saliva. The total disbelief and bewilderment of that moment has never left me. Yes, I had signed a consent form to say it 'could' be a consequence of surgery, but no significance was given to it at the time of signing. Not for a second did I think it would be relevant to me. Following a subsequent tricky experience with aspiration pneumonia following an altercation with soup, a feeding tube became my new best friend. Nearly 10 years on, with steely determination and a newfound appreciation of all things edible, I am happy to say that I am no longer reliant on a tube and have a relatively unassuming, non-choking relationship with food. Albeit soft food, but nonetheless nutrition that no longer shoots out my nose like some weird party trick. Several things have helped me get to this point. A fantastic speech therapist (think they are called speech pathologist in the US) and a dietitian were tasked with showing me how to turn my head 90 degrees to the affected side and to 'swallow, cough, swallow' in order to protect my airway. They became adept at wearing an apron and wellington boots during my barium swallow procedures, as my reputation for decorating the room with barium became iconic! Tucking my chin on my chest whilst swallowing also worked well. Although at times, I would forget to close my lips properly and the offending food would end up in my lap! Iced smoothies also stimulated my throat and thickening agents made getting liquids down easier. I

became a firm acquaintance of my blender and gave house room to seemingly hundreds of bottles of chocolate and mocha protein shakes. I quickly learnt that you could freeze the shakes too for added luxury! I also developed a massive respect for my airway and appreciated just how precarious the process of propelling food downwards truly is. I pined for salad leaves (and still do), which was odd as I was never that enamored with greenery when I could eat them! Most of all, I had an unrelenting determination to learn to swallow again, however impossible that seemed in the early days. Tears of frustration were slowly replaced with tears of joy—I embraced all the support groups I could muster and no wacky ideas or alternative therapies were dismissed. I had cognitive behavior therapy and counseling to adjust to my new challenges and learnt to laugh in the face of adversity. The journey with dysphagia is incredibly hard and lonely, as food is such an integral part of life and something that is taken for granted. Swallowing still regularly throws me a curve ball, but on a positive note, my resulting throat numbness has made Covid swab testing an absolute breeze. Silver linings and all that! I wish you well with your journey. Know that wherever you are, you are never alone."

—Julia Proporowicz

"'Empathy' is the term I associate myself with nowadays. Living in a developed country, we are prone to a lot of power-cuts. These blackouts mean that the grinder doesn't work, which in turn means that I have to either be content with a bowl of curd or a yogurt or a pudding. In this time of coronavirus crisis, even these desserts are a rarity. People often enquire about the diet I follow as I completely transformed into a thin person. I retort by hard laughter and walk off. They say that they are jealous of my slim physique and that they want to be in my place, but I really don't want anyone in this world to go through my exhaustive ailment. Dysphagia taught me resilience and perseverance. I *am now a completely different person, who is devoid of anger, greed, selfishness, and prejudice. Being a teacher, it's my duty to educate and positively transform my students, and I sincerely feel that now I am truly practicing what I preach to everyone. The following are some of my coping strategies:*

• I developed pureed food/soft food recipes that nourish me throughout the day and satisfy my taste buds too. I also refer to lot of dysphagia cookbooks that are available on Amazon.

• I consider dysphagia as a blessing as it has given me an opportunity to be unique.

• I am also getting lot of emotional support from my family, friends and well-wishers.

• I don't feel lonely anymore as I am always surrounded by lot of curious SLPs & ENTs trying to cure me.

• I found a purpose for my life, i.e., apart from developing my own semi-solid delicacies, I have also found many transitional solid foods that can be easily melted immediately after chewing. My book has benefited more than 1,000 dysphagia patients in India. All is Well!

• I serve food to the needy every day. Needy includes beggars, street animals, etc. Seeing their happiness gives a lot of energy. I even found Love!

• I pray three times a day to the God of food & Health in my religion. The Secret!

• Sharing my predicament helped me a lot as I was received very well at whichever place I go taking into account my eating habits.

• I enjoy every day. I'm working in the day. Evenings I go jogging. Weekends means movies, restaurants, and chilling at the beach. I spoke to the chefs in the restaurants that I regularly visit so that they modify my food before serving. I try to never miss out on any enjoyment that normal people have. I enjoy beverages as much as I can. I consider bad days as body cleansing days. I live my life to the fullest, getting happiness in minute progresses and developments in my swallow every day. Positivity is most important!"

—Dr. Challa Krishnaveer Abhishek

Soft Skills Trainer of Andhra University & Founder-Secretary of Centre for Emotional Education Society. In his ebook *Emotional Linguistic Therapy & Dysphagia*, Dr. Abhlshek shares his story as well as tips and tools for others going through this. krishnava.elt@gmail.com.

"I have dysphagia for many years. I notice or am aware of the fact that I get very angry when I hear people complain about food or their diets. I am also sad when I see people eating—all normal in this situation with so much lack. I also realized that the anger and nasty things said under my breath do not serve me. That it is only weakening me and causing me pain. So now when I feel the anger at them and resentment I try to refocus or think of something I am grateful for. I was in the park yesterday and heard a woman bitch and moan about her limited diet to lose weight and I heard the familiar nasty comments start to gather in my mind. I immediately focused on something I was grateful for—being in the park— breathing. Seeing cherry blossoms. Anger is normal. Grief is a normal part of this, but I know now that the resentments only build as long as I continue to focus on what I do not have or cannot do."

John G.

"I've been doing TV dinners and blended each of the items up and put it back into the tray for my husband who has dysphagia from a stroke and a brain disorder. I've been doing this for two years straight and use thicker for liquid foods and beverages as well. If you want to have a burrito just put it in a blender. For us, I use a Magic Bullet and add a little bit of water for moisture and blend until it's mushy. Or French toasts, add a little bit of milk and blend until it's moist enough. You want it like mashed potatoes texture. I do that with fish sticks, chicken patties, pot pies, and such. I just learned how to make a puree PB&J. It's like you're making a PB&J Sandwich—then cut them in small squares like bite size, then add in to a Magic Bullet, then add a little bit of milk, then blend. It will be pudding like in texture. Just don't add too much liquid."

—Deborah G.,
Caregiver for her husband

" I know everyone is different but I know from my experience that just because I am on a level 5 there are things that I can't tolerate. Adapt and overcome has become my motto."

—Sue Boyce

"My husband bought me a converter for our vehicle so I can take my NutriBullet RX or Vitamix with us. I run outside, blend up my food, and run back in to enjoy being in the restaurant."

—Wendy

"Food without texture can be frustrating but you can replace texture by finding flavors that make your mouth happy. Juicers and blenders can be the best appliances in your kitchen if you're

willing to try new things."

—Amy J. Eger

"Pinterest has a ton of recipes for dysphagia. I started a board on it for my husband. He had chemo and 35 rounds of radiation for Nasopharyngeal Carcinoma way back in 2004/2005 and lost some of his taste and all of his saliva. Now he is having increased difficulty swallowing and spent two weeks in the hospital. He was terribly sick and they thought it was lung cancer. It turns out he has been aspirating his food and liquids into his lungs and has been going on for a long time due to choking. Now, all he can have is thickened liquids and pureed foods, and it seems to be helping. He does like a hot dog or sausage pureed. I toss in a toasted hot dog roll in the blender with mustard, relish and a little milk. The other night we were having baked beans on the side so I tossed them in too. It seemed to make it smoother. He ate it all. I also have been freezing portions of all meals that I make and puree, so some nights are easier. It takes a lot of prep work to make meals for him and a lot of dishes, so freezing the left over portions is helpful."

—Diane Martin

pinterest.ca/dmartin1965/dysphagia-recipes

"Know that the pain of hunger can be intense for the first few months while your body adjusts, but the hunger pain eases. Feeling depressed is normal for this condition especially in the first few months as you mentally, physically and socially adapt to your changed relationship with food. People don't realize our relationship with food touches so many areas of our lives until they suddenly lose the ability to eat. It's a really difficult journey and I felt like I was dying when it first started with the rapid

weight loss, pain, medical procedures and lack of answers. I still don't have a cause determined, so I have just learned to deal with it for now. I had not really considered that someone who has not had a stroke or a disability could suddenly lose an important function in their bodies, but then it happened to me.

Do not lose sight that it is possible to adapt, and things can get easier over time. Focusing on or finding other areas of your life that brings you joy is important, and it can help to find a trauma informed counselor who can help you do this. It's been a really hard slog and I think it's important to validate the tough parts too, but it needs to be balanced with hope and encouragement. It's the only way I've gone through all this and still managed to work, raise my kids and function. And of course, invest in a good blender and make smoothies with a nutritional supplement to help sustain your physical health." -

—Tracy Roser

"I have swallowing and eating challenges due to head and neck cancer. I loved food pre illness and treatment. Afterwards I found it easier to go to counseling and have a change of mindset on how I viewed food and eating. Puree and similar options are not for me. I live off high calorie protein shakes. Sometimes I eat soup and taste things here and there. Personally it was too emotional and off putting to puree. I suggest not being afraid of changing the way you eat and view food. It is a hard road. I did two years of counseling due to food grief. Food is everywhere and everything revolves around food and drink. We have to find ways to conquer and adapt. All my thoughts and prayers to others going through this too."

—Jennifer Allen Perkins

"If you blend in some olive oil to soups you get a lot of calories from the oil alone. Pureed broccoli cheese soup is calorific. Try to incorporate healthy fats into everything for calories if needed. My favorites are avocado and olive oil. Pureed lentil soups is an excellent source of protein, fiber and calories."

—Matt Armitage

"I'm presuming I'm stating the obvious, but the Dysphagia Foods & Recipes Group on Facebook has been amazing and a big part of my 'getting through each day. I have also been trying a few things from this resource book. Last night I watched funny clips on You Tube. I was laughing until with tears rolling down my face and I then had the best sleep in weeks. It is wonderful. The simple things in life we forget about. I feel like a child again. These emotions are squashed down during survival mode but it is what we really need while in survival mode."

- Sally Gillespie

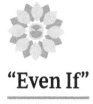

"Even If"

I wrote the following piece years ago. It has been viewed over 25,000 times on Elephant Journal *and has been published in the book by Amy Scher,* Lessons from Lyme Disease, Chronic Fatigue and Fibromyalgia. *It is also on the NFOSD website under the personal stories section. The most heartfelt letters I get are from people with dysphagia who have brought this piece of writing to their psychologist or to family members to show them what it is like for them to live with this condition. I received a letter only this week from a woman in New Zealand who said that her boyfriend was better able to understand what she was going through after reading the following piece. I have included it in this book just for that reason.*

"Even If."

Adam and I are standing outside a Chinese restaurant at night, waiting for a bus.

The distinctive smell of Szechwan cuisine escaping from the restaurant onto the street surrounds me. It fills my nose and sends a signal to my brain that I am hungry. I start to cry. I am standing on Second Avenue crying because I can't eat.

Adam sees me crying and without a word, he holds my hand. The smell of the food is so strong and exquisite that he need not question why I am crying—he knows.

There is this heavy grief within for not being able to eat normally, for not being able to socialize around food or sit at a table with others breaking bread. I have tried over the years to sit at tables while others eat, but I end up crying or making the people around me feel uncomfortable. I bring my liquified concoction, but often noise and

85

movement in the restaurant is too much—even swallowing my drink in public can be too overwhelming to my nervous system.

All my energy and effort and concentration go into swallowing. The swallowing therapist at NYU told me this is normal, and that any distraction can take away from the focus of eating, which needs all my concentration. What once required no thought or concentration now requires thought, concentration, and a lot of prayers. I marvel at others eating.

I once stared at a woman briskly walking down the street—her yoga bag hanging from her back as she ate an apple. She looked at me, most likely wondering why I was staring. I stared because to walk and eat at the same time is a wonder to me, as if I just saw the most amazing magic act right in front of me. I see her take a bite and then another, and the apple slowly disappears. I wonder if she knows how miraculous it all is, but I am sure she does not. I know when I could eat I did not know how miraculous it was either.

I watch in awe a man cycling down First Avenue on his bike while eating a slice of pizza. "Wow!" I say aloud. Biking and eating at the same time seems incredible, and yet he does it with ease. I watch kids as they eat cupcakes while they walk or gobble up bagels as they play. I see how they can even skip while eating, as if it is the most natural thing in the world. I guess it is. These are things I never noticed when I could eat.

In Manhattan, there is a restaurant on every block, often more than one. The smells of cuisine from all over the world lingers outside of the incredible number of restaurants in the borough: Indian, Italian, Chinese, Israeli, Burmese, Thai, Soul food. Often all the aromas join together as if in a dance. Each smell pokes me in the gut and my heart. "Here, look what you can't have, Julia," they say to me. "Look what is not for you!"

Food is everywhere. Often, when I smell the heavenly aromas coming out of restaurants, I hear my stomach talking to me, not understanding. If my mouth is salivating, why then do I not go into the restaurant and get that piece of pizza? I can't. I can't swallow it.

"Go in there and order that piece of white pizza with onions," says my stomach, which, for some reason, sounds like a grumpy old man. "That guy in there is eating a slice? What's wrong with you, kid?"

How do I explain this to my stomach? I can hardly understand all this myself.

"I know you want that pizza with all of your heart or gut," I silently reply. "But the transit to get it to you is faulty right now. There is a glitch in the system."

All I hear back is my stomach making hungry gurgling sounds. The smell of pizza does that to my stomach.

There is shock, and many times, I have said to myself, "Okay, Julia, this is what happened: You had this accident—or this virus or mold infection damaged your nerves or brain or your neck—and then you lost your ability to swallow." But it still makes no sense, because it is so odd and so completely unfair.

Living with a debilitating chronic illness for so many years was hard enough, but this? I was angry with God. I thought I got back my ability to swallow and that it would last forever, and I worked so hard! Did I climb up this mountain just to fall to the bottom again? "Why did you take this away again?" I asked, as if I might get an answer or could know the whys. Even the doctors don't know why this happened to me. It could be a virus, could be an infection, could be brain damage. It could be . . . fill in the blank.

In every article about dysphagia, they write of the depression caused by being unable to be part of social life. Most of social life is food: breaking bread, sharing a meal. The loss of that connection—that social connection—can be devastating. It has been heartbreaking for me too.

I go to NYU Langone Hospital to get another barium swallow test. The nurse and doctor watch from the X-ray room, and I can see their faces through the glass partition as I swallow concoctions of chalky barium. The nurse, who reminds me of a blonde Betty Boop character, is trying to be funny. "I've seen worse," she says.

A week later, my neurologist enters her office with the test results in her hands. The look on her face is one of helplessness and no answers. You have a big problem, she says. That was it. There was no, "You have a problem, Ms. Tuchman, and this is how we are going to fix it—two hours in the operating room and then pizza!" Cheers and applause. Joyous cinematic music used for the life-changing scene begins to play in the background. This would be fixed in no time. No, none of that. They have no cure and no answers. Neurology is a specialty field with no answers, I have learned.

While walking down a Manhattan street, I stop at the window of a cozy-looking Chinese restaurant. I watch a family eating at a large table, laughing and smiling, and I am brought back in my mind to my childhood when my parents would bring my siblings and me to Tung Sing. We would eat the wonderful food, while the staff would often have fights in the kitchen—throwing plates of food and arguing in Chinese. It was all wonderful and magical, but far more than I even knew then.

I did not know about such things then, such as not being able to swallow food or severe illness. I knew Tung Sing was the best. I loved going to Tung Sing where egg rolls, spare ribs, and those crunchy fried noodles were always waiting for me. I watched this family now through the window, my mind taking me back to Tung Sing so many years ago and the feeling of family and laughter. I wanted that again. I snapped out of the memory of ghosts of Chinese meals past and continued walking on.

Once, I watched a couple through the window of a restaurant holding hands while eating. I envied them. There were lovely plates full of food in front of them, and they were smiling. Adam and I were together at this time, and I would have given anything to be sitting in a restaurant with him eating a meal like that.

I went with Adam to a Thai restaurant for his birthday. I brought my liquefied soup and asked the woman who owned the restaurant for a bowl. She seemed upset, as if my not eating her food was a personal snub. I tried to explain, but she became even more confused. Adam ate, and I tried to get my liquid soup down. We tried to pretend, but I could feel the pain in my heart, and I could see the sadness in his eyes. This was one thing we could not share.

Focusing on the swimming, exotic fish in the fish tank to get my mind off the Thai food smells, I focused on my gratitude for being able to be in the restaurant and share in his special day. I focused on the surroundings. I focused on being able to see and smell the food and to talk. All miracles. But I felt left out—an outsider from this important part of life, this physical need, this social need—and, worst of all, this might be for life.

"But you are alive," my father will often remind me. "Where there is life there is hope," he says to me often. "It came back once before," he says. "It can come back again." He is right—Mila, the Holocaust survivor who lives at his assisted living facility, holds my hand when I first meet her and tells me, "If your eyes are still open, there is hope." I listen to her—she would know.

I have been at an abyss many times in this journey, when it felt there was nothing left. There was emptiness so deep and grief so wide that it filled all of me and extended out into the world I saw. There are silent screams that fill me, and this was one of those days. I did not want to live in deprivation any longer.

I walk by a restaurant on one of those days—I am on the other side of the windowpane separating me from the diners, and I pass by one table after another filled with people eating lunch. A woman about my age eats a grilled cheese sandwich, a favorite of mine as a kid. I used to put French fries in the sandwich with ketchup. People would laugh at my odd combination, but I loved it.

I am brought back to my childhood and to my days when eating was effortless and life seemed sweeter. I begin to cry. I instinctively put my hand up to my throat in a loving gentle swoop and say aloud, "I love you, Julia." My voice sounds kind, like a mother comforting her child. With each table I pass, I say, "I love you, Julia, I love you." Another table with a family eating—"I love you, Julia"—tears fall as this kindness engulfs me. I was starving for this loving kindness to myself as much as I was hungry for food.

This was not a planned, "I love you, Julia," after reading a self-help book or even a conscious decision. It was not what I was supposed to do, or what I was told to do. It came from the depths of my soul, spoke to my heart, then to my voice box and brain as well, and out of my mouth with no conscious thought. An "I love you" escaped from me into the Manhattan air and then back to my own ears. I was speaking to myself and to that dark emptiness and desperation I felt draining any will to go on. I was filling myself up. I was nourishing myself.

I had lost so much in all these years. I had lost so much but I had this— the gentle touch to my throat and the kind words to myself in spite of it all. There was power in that. There is something about invisible disability that is doubly hurtful. Nobody sees it or understands it, and so they judge.

When I told my neurologist I did not want to live like this, he told me, "I don't blame you." He was truthful, but these words were not helpful to hear. I would have loved to hear, "Lay your burdens down. I understand. I can help you." But I knew only I could offer myself that comfort.

I have judged myself, and I have beaten myself up over and over, as if I were somehow responsible for all the years of illness and seemingly endless knock-downs. But on that day, when I passed those people eating and touched my throat, speaking kind, loving words to myself—that choice was the healing.

Still, allowing myself to grieve is healing me. I don't think I permitted myself to feel the grief for years. Instead, my focus was on getting from point A to point B, and which doctor would help me eat again. It was the way I coped. But I am learning to allow myself to feel the feelings as they arise.

There are many books on how to be happy or how to have this or that fixed in 10 days. What if we accept what is and allow those feelings that are so scary to us to come up? Sometimes I am fearful it will overtake me, because there is so much of it, but I still allow it. When I feel grief now, I sit with it and don't fight it. What a relief to not fight. I allow the feelings to come and go like waves—no resistance or judgment.

Last week, I arrived early for a doctor's appointment, and I sat with my eyes closed in the waiting room to rest. The secretaries were talking for a half hour about which restaurant they wanted to go to for a large family get-together. They mentioned every type of food and every type of restaurant available in New York. One was eating McDonald's and another was eating a sandwich as they discussed their plans. I had my thermos of protein shake. I was surprised at how neutral I felt. I was hearing them talk, but not attached to what they said. I let the words flow over me and through me.

"You really want to test me, God," I said aloud to the ceiling of the empty waiting room as they continued talking about my favorite meals. I was assuming God was in the ceiling of a doctor's office. I am certain the ceiling of waiting rooms hear many prayers.

I touched my throat and sent myself love. I also sent blessings to my liquefied food and went to a place of gratitude for it. It was getting easier. Somehow it was getting easier in the acceptance of it all and the allowing. I even gave myself acknowledgement for how far I have come and how these lessons in self-love were healing me.

There is a flow in these sacred moments of self-love and acceptance—like riding waves. There are losses and regrets that have crushed me, or so I thought, but I have gotten up again, even after being toppled by those waves that seemed far too big and heartbreaking. And I rise again and again, with, "I love you, Julia."

"I love you, Julia," I say as I touch my throat. "I love you even if you can't eat normally. I love you even if this is forever. I love you even if this all heals tomorrow. I even love you if this never heals."

I touch my throat and send it love. That I can do. I can do that.

Julia Tuchman Is a CTA coach and consultant who offers one-on-one sessions for those with chronic illness and dysphagia. If you are interested in supportive counseling sessions, you can email Julia at julia@juliatuchman.com

Amazon Smile is a program that allows some revenue from your purchases on Amazon to go to a charity of your choice. The NFOSD (National Foundation of Swallowing Disorders) is one of the charities. The foundation has been a life raft for so many with this disorder. I have chosen them as my Amazon Smile charity. It's a simple way for the NFOSD to raise money. When you shop on Amazon, enter the site via smile.amazon.com in order to support NFOSD at no extra cost to you. Please note that the NFOSD is listed as "National Foundation of Swallowingdisorders" with no space between the words "swallowing" and "disorders."

Acknowledgments

For and in memory of my dear parents Kenneth (Moe) and Esther who were (and are) the unwavering unconditional love in my life that sustains me. My Mom was able to read the earliest version of this book, and encouraged me to get it out there because it would "help so many people". She was a true healer and "helper" in this world. This is for you Mom.

Thank you to the following: Robin Herman, who always had my back and taught me how to be NY tough—whose guidance and support I still feel from the other side. Athena Groumoutis, (my Canadian sister) whose friendship and support has been a blessing in my life. Also thank you to Adam Wolinsky, Helene Goldberg, Rita Lloyd, Ron Jaffe, Dr. Teresa Ashman, Laura Dumbrava, Lynn Auerbach, Dr. Netin Sethi and Dr. Robert Frey. Gratitude for my talented and creative brother Mark, who created the cover for this book and did all the formatting. My sister Paula T. Weiss who edited and Heather Rose Ryan who also graciously edited and supported this project.

And thank you to Tricia Reilly Bowles, who I have never met, but still flew across the Atlantic one night to remind me to begin to write.

Made in United States
North Haven, CT
03 January 2023

30572278R00061